Advance praise for *Unblinded*

"*Unblinded* is a once-in-a-lifetime story, a journey through darkness and light, love and loss, awakening and discovery. Its pages take us, at once, on a remarkable true adventure and into the heart and mind of a most extraordinary individual. A beautifully written and inspiring tale, and a reminder to us all about what really matters."

–ROBERT KURSON, *New York Times*
bestselling author of *Crashing Through, Shadow*
Divers, Pirate Hunters **and** *Rocket Men*

"*Unblinded* tells a remarkable story of sudden blindness, new vision, and sight regained. It offers great insight into the nature of reality—that which we perceive and that which we create for ourselves."

–ISAAC LIDSKY, *New York Times*
bestselling author of *Eyes Wide Open*

"*Unblinded* provides honest, profound insight into the emotional trauma that occurs when vision is lost and the path forward in life cannot be seen."

–LISSA POINCENOT, National Leber's
Hereditary Optic Neuropathy Advocate

"Miracles can happen from the inside out. In *Unblinded*, Traci Medford-Rosow leads us through the wondrous story of one man's experience of overcoming blindness. *Unblinded* takes the reader on a fascinating, behind-the-scenes tour of what went on during those years of darkness and how Kevin Coughlin, after battling alcoholism, loneliness, prejudice, and perhaps most of all himself, emerges as a man of wisdom and sight."

–ANN CAMPANELLA, Award-winning and bestselling author of *Motherhood: Lost and Found*

"*Unblinded:* A tale about overcoming personal tragedy risks sentimentality. *Unblinded* offers instead a sightless perspective on reality that could engage a physicist."

–PROF. NEIL J. SULLIVAN, Author: *The Prometheus Bomb* and *The Dodgers Move West*

"In *Unblinded*, you will see how what we say and the way we think does become our reality. What an eye opener reading *Unblinded* was for me. The struggles with alcoholism, life, and being blind caused Kevin to make a mental as well as physical paradigm shift into willing his life back to wellness. Kevin begins to realize that as he muddles through this battle, he is a living, walking miracle."

–Readers' Favorite, VERNITA NAYLOR, Five Star Review

Unblinded

Unblinded

One Man's Courageous Journey through Darkness to Sight

Traci Medford-Rosow and Kevin Coughlin

NEW YORK

LONDON • NASHVILLE • MELBOURNE • VANCOUVER

Unblinded

One Man's Courageous Journey Through Darkness to Sight

Published in New York, New York, by Morgan James Publishing. Morgan James is a trademark of Morgan James, LLC. www.MorganJamesPublishing.com

The Morgan James Speakers Group can bring authors to your live event. For more information or to book an event visit The Morgan James Speakers Group at www.TheMorganJamesSpeakersGroup.com.

The information in this book is not intended to diagnose or treat any medical condition nor to serve as a substitute for informed medical advice or care. All events are true. Some of the names of the people and organizations have been changed to protect their privacy.

The following are registered trademarks:
New York Times, Fresca, Sears, Lacoste, Levi's, Waldbaums, Ralph Lauren, Tommy Hilfiger, Calvin Klein, Vans, Bang and Olufsen, Canon, LL Bean, Swatch, Rolling Stone, Seeing Eye, Saks Fifth Avenue, Mutual of America, Stoli, JAWS, Barneys, Ferragamo, Astroland, Cyclone.

ISBN 9781683507826 paperback
ISBN 9781683507840 case laminate
ISBN 9781683507833 eBook
Library of Congress Control Number: 2017915232

Cover and Interior Design by:
Chris Treccani
www.3dogcreative.net

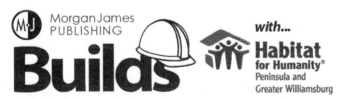

In an effort to support local communities, raise awareness and funds, Morgan James Publishing donates a percentage of all book sales for the life of each book to Habitat for Humanity Peninsula and Greater Williamsburg.

Get involved today! Visit
www.MorganJamesBuilds.com

Kevin Coughlin wakes up one morning in 1997 and cannot read the newspaper. Even the bold headlines are fuzzy. Kevin has no idea that he is carrying a rare genetic disorder: Leber's Hereditary Optic Neuropathy. Within five days he is blind.

The tragedy of his sudden blindness is exacerbated by the fact that Kevin is a serious amateur photographer and lover of the visual arts. Every aspect of his life is plunged into unbearable darkness.

Kevin's loss of sight initiates an exploration of his internal world. After decades of heavy drinking, he embarks on the long and difficult road to sobriety. He discovers the powerful effect of his thoughts and spoken words. He chooses to focus on gratitude for what he has rather than on anger at what he has lost.

In a world of darkness, he sees how to be kinder to himself and others. He becomes an activist for the blind as only a person who once had eyesight could and is instrumental in establishing New York City's first blind advocacy program.

Fifteen years later, Kevin catches what seems to be a glimpse of light in his bathroom mirror. Kevin's is the only documented case in the world of a non-medically assisted regeneration of the optic nerve.

Over the next three years, Kevin chronicles the daily progress—the euphoria and the agonizing setbacks. It is from those journal entries and deeply moving conversations with Kevin that author Traci Medford-Rosow has shaped Kevin's remarkable story.

Unblinded is a story of miracles within miracles that will leave the reader wondering what lies behind the reality we think we see.

Author's Note to Readers:

This is a true story of one man's remarkable battle to regain his eyesight after suddenly losing it to a rare genetic disorder. All events are true, however, the names of some of the people and organizations have been changed to protect their privacy.

I first learned of Kevin Coughlin on Easter morning 2016. My husband returned from walking our two dogs, breathless with excitement—a blind man in our New York City neighborhood had miraculously regained his sight!

Kevin was looking for someone to write his story, and I agreed to do it. Kevin kept a journal chronicling the return of his vision. A selected entry appears after each chapter. However, the entire unedited journal can be found in the appendix.

As our weekly work progressed, it soon became clear that I was witnessing a man who had become "unblind" not only in his vision, but in his soul, as well.

Acknowledgements:

I would like to thank Kevin Coughlin for trusting me to write his amazing story, and in so doing, hopefully sharing it with many others. A special thanks to my husband, Joel Rosow, for his patience in helping us shape the story and in his tireless review of numerous drafts. To my developmental editor, Richard Kelley, who always knows what the story is even before I know it myself, you are indeed my Max Perkins, Editor-of-Genius. To Sarah Saffian, my teacher at the Sarah Lawrence Writing Institute, author of *Ithaka: A Daughter's Memoir of Being Found* and copy editor par none, thank you for teaching me how to create the "tick-tock" of my stories. To my publicist extraordinaire, Laura Ponticello, award-winning and bestselling author of *The Art of Self Transformation* and *Live the Life of Your Dreams*, thank you for helping to spread my stories and for teaching me the fine art of elucidating their transformative nature. To my proofreader, Danielle Gasparro, thank you for catching all those hard-to-find typos! A special thanks to my friends and family who read early drafts, including Jeff Worron, Phyllis Reiss, Rita Selby, Alan Saly, Tarja Antonetti, Joan Rosow, and my law partner, Peter Richardson—your input, suggestions and encouragement are essential. Last, but not least, a heartfelt thanks to my editors, cover designers and publishers at Morgan James.

Dedication:

To Sister Dolores and Jim.

For inspiring me by living their lives with dignity and grace.
Most important, for showing me that blindness had the
potential to be an empowering force rather than a limiting one.

–KEVIN COUGHLIN

The wound is where the Light enters you.
–RUMI

CONTENTS

PROLOGUE

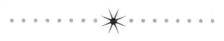

Friday, June 17, 2016

For a brief moment, Kevin did not know where he was. An eerie predawn silence blanketed the summer air. It was four o'clock in the morning. The birds were still quiet; the dawn chorus had not yet begun. Elias, his dog, begrudgingly stirred when Kevin sat up in bed.

Kevin felt his way through the unfamiliar house, trying to be as quiet as possible so he wouldn't wake his friend. He made his way up the flight of stairs and out onto the back deck.

The house was perched on a cliff overlooking a lake. Kevin wanted to enjoy the rising sun—to experience the warmth as it touched his upturned face.

The air smelled fresh—if a bit too sweet from the abundance of floral scents competing for his attention. Nevertheless, it was a welcome relief from the cloying, and often putrid, summer air in the city. He could hear waves gently lapping against the boat dock below and the first faint, distant quacks of ducks. Kevin found a deck chair and lowered himself into it. Elias settled down next to him.

As dawn approached, Kevin searched for the warmest spot on the horizon; he knew that was where the sun would peek up first. Something above caught his attention, distracting his gaze. He raised his head and forced his eyes upward.

Kevin began to cry, although he had no idea why.

At first, he thought the faint lights in the sky were something teasing his optic nerve. He wasn't sure if he was hallucinating or merely remembering what the night sky looked like right before daybreak. Suddenly, Kevin's brain caught up with his emotions. As he steadied his eyes, he could see the reason for his unexplained tears—the hazy outline of tiny stars twinkling in the fading darkness.

Kevin hurried inside, stumbled back down the stairs to his room, and picked up his journal. He wanted to make the latest entry while the emotional sensation was still fresh in his memory.

I am seated in a wicker rocker facing Lake Mahopac. The delicious stillness is suddenly interrupted by spasms of joy-filled tears. After a momentary lapse, it becomes evident why I am crying. For the first time in nineteen years. I am seeing a star-filled sky.

PART ONE

DESCENT INTO DARKNESS

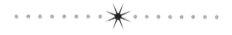

1997-2001

"Darkness cannot drive out darkness, only light can do that."
–MARTIN LUTHER KING, JR.

CHAPTER 1

Blue Eyes

Saturday, February 15, 1997

Kevin couldn't shake an ominous feeling that had been nagging him for two days.

He glanced at the liquor cabinet. It was too early to have a drink, even by his liberal definition of when cocktail hour began.

He distracted himself from that thought by picking up the *New York Times*. And there it was again. The same blurriness he'd experienced two days earlier at work. He was doing some research for his latest grant proposal when he noticed he was unable to read an article he'd pulled off the reference shelf. The words were blurry. Soft. Out of focus.

He hadn't been too concerned about it at the time. He thought he was just tired after a long day at the office, and anyway, it was a problem easily solved. He made the short trip to the Xerox machine and enlarged the print.

But this was Saturday morning in his own home. And he'd had a good night's sleep. His eyes were not in the least strained from a long day at work. Kevin wondered if he needed glasses. He started to blink rapidly, but his efforts produced little, if any, improvement in his vision. He put the newspaper on his coffee table and headed for the bathroom. He washed and dried his face, paying particular attention to his eyes. As he returned to his living room, he glanced out the window. It seemed foggy outside. At the same moment, he heard the weather report on the television—bitterly cold with abundant sunshine.

Kevin couldn't dwell on it for long, however. He was going to visit his parents on Long Island. Walking across town to Penn Station was uneventful. Kevin had done it so many times; the ten blocks from his apartment on Lexington and 37th posed no problem, even though his vision was still blurry.

He didn't need to read the information board—his train always departed from track eighteen. He headed toward it. Once on the train, he sat down in his usual seat next to the window and made himself comfortable. It was a forty-minute trip out to Mineola.

He hadn't brought the newspaper with him. There was no point in reminding himself about the eyesight issue more than necessary. Anyway, he was still convinced it was no big deal. It was, he thought once again, as simple as needing glasses. After all, he was thirty-six, and many of his friends had purchased their first pair a decade earlier.

His mother was sitting in her car when the train pulled into the station. Kevin could always count on her waiting in the parking lot—even on those evenings when he'd fallen asleep on the train and missed his stop.

Ruth Liesenberg Coughlin was a nurturing and devoted mother. She was a private duty nurse by training which suited her personality well. A kind and loving woman, not only to her family but also to her friends, she was adored by everyone. Kevin never failed to be in awe of, or grateful for, her loyalty. On the other hand, Kevin felt that his father, Walter J. Coughlin, an accountant by profession, was somewhat emotionally distant. Nevertheless, Kevin appreciated the fact that he'd been a good provider for his family and a faithful husband to Ruth.

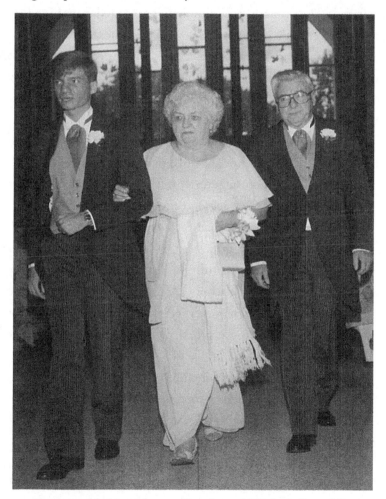

Kevin with his parents, Ruth and Walter Coughlin

Kevin was the youngest of three children. His sister, Kathy, and brother, John, were ten and eight years older. The gap made him feel like an only child for much of his youth, especially once Kathy and John left for college.

Kevin was overweight from the age of five to fifteen. As a result, he lacked confidence and was socially awkward. He had few, if any, close friends. His primary social interactions resulted from his reluctant participation in Little League and his weekly attendance at mass.

In his sophomore year of high school, Kevin decided to transform himself. He went on a diet consisting of tuna fish and Fresca, started working out, and lost forty pounds. Miraculously, as he lost girth he gained height. He grew four inches taller.

Kevin, the short and chubby one, had disappeared along with the fat boy clothes his mother bought for him in the Husky Shop at Sears. Fashionable Levi's and Lacoste polo shirts took their place. He became a tall, slender, green-eyed hunk just in time for college.

Kevin and his mother returned to the family home—the same blue Cape Cod house where he'd grown up. He always loved the back yard; it was one of the deepest and flattest in the neighborhood. It had been a great place for parties in high school. After years of feeling unaccepted, Kevin had gained a modicum of respect from his peers by junior year, even though he suspected it was primarily because of the party venue he was able to provide.

His parents' bedroom was on the first floor; the kids' rooms were upstairs. This provided a fair measure of privacy, which came in handy when Kevin wanted to crank up his radio or record player and listen to his favorite Elton John and Billy Joel albums.

Their neighborhood, like many others on Long Island that were part of the post-war building boom, was built on an old potato field. There were three models to choose from—a Cape Cod, split level, or ranch. This was a big deal in the 1950's. Most of the other neighborhoods in the area had only one choice.

After a quick bite to eat, Kevin set off for Waldbaum's to do his parents' weekly grocery shopping, a chore he had taken over after his father's stroke five years earlier. Kevin stuffed his mother's list into his pocket, and, as usual, assured her he'd be back soon. He always looked forward to his trips to Waldbaum's. In contrast to the city's grocery stores, Waldbaum's was clean and bright. The food was organized, making his task an easy and pleasant one. He knew where to go for the usual items: fruit, vegetables, meat, milk, and the two 12-packs of diet soda his father loved.

That day, however, the store seemed to lack its customary brightness. The colors appeared as muted shades of gray that matched the mood of the winter day. The oranges, lemons and selection of colorful vegetables that filled meticulously arranged display stands looked washed out.

In this dull light, Kevin had a problem reading the grocery list. He stood in the produce department studying it for several minutes, willing the words to come into focus. Short of asking someone in the store to walk around with him like a personal shopper, he knew there was only one thing to do. He would have to return home to ask his mother to read the list aloud to him or write it larger.

Kevin was not eager to do this as he knew it would alarm her. His own internal warning lights were flashing in his head, yet he continued to subdue them with his self-diagnosis that he needed nothing more than a pair of reading glasses.

As he predicted, when Kevin walked in the front door empty-handed, his mother's tone of voice confirmed that she was worried.

"What are you doing back so soon? Where are the groceries?"

"I'm sorry, but I can't read the grocery list, mom. Can you please rewrite it and make it bigger?"

Ruth let out a sound that was somewhat of a grunt mixed with concern and disappeared into the kitchen for another piece of scrap paper. Kevin followed her.

As he sat at the kitchen table waiting for his mother to rewrite the list, he realized that he couldn't see the color of his mother's vivid blue eyes. Or the details of her face, which was remarkably unlined for someone in her seventies.

Kevin didn't say anything. He didn't want to alarm her further. He took the rewritten grocery list from his mother's outstretched hand and glanced at it. He still couldn't make out the words. Reluctant to cause additional worry but unable to return to Waldbaum's with the proffered list, he asked again.

"Mom, would you please make the words a bit bigger? I guess I'm tired from being out late last night, and I'm still having a hard time reading the list."

Kevin hadn't been out late the night before—in fact he hadn't been out at all. Ruth was no longer able to hide her growing concern.

"You need to see an eye doctor first thing next week," she said adamantly. "Please promise me you'll make an appointment when you get back to the city."

Kevin nodded his agreement. He then cast his eyes over the new grocery list with its oversized letters written in black felt-tipped pen on a yellow legal pad. His mother gave him an anxious look. He simply touched her shoulder and headed back to Waldbaum's to complete his shopping.

Kevin didn't discuss his eyesight with his father that day, but he overheard his mother talking to him.

"Walter, Kevin is having problems with his eyesight, and I'm worried."

Kevin walked out of earshot of the conversation. He didn't want to hear the rest. Kevin could no longer convince himself, much less his parents, that his poor eyesight could be corrected with a pair of reading glasses.

* * *

By the time Kevin returned to his apartment that evening, he knew something was very wrong. It was as if the lights were being dimmed. If he couldn't understand what was going on, he could at least numb it.

He reached for the vodka.

He poured himself a full glass leaving only enough room for a splash of cranberry juice. He paused when he took the container from the fridge.

Something was strange.

He picked up a carton of orange juice. He blinked rapidly, shook his head, and looked once more at the drink containers, comparing them side-by-side. He shook his head, blinked again and rubbed his eyes.

Kevin was no longer able to see colors.

SELECTED JOURNAL ENTRY:

August 14, 2013—entering the bathroom at 1 a.m., I am perplexed and mesmerized by the reflection of light in my medicine cabinet mirror. I think I must be dreaming or imagining it.

CHAPTER 2

Liquid Confidence

Sunday, February 16-Tuesday February 18, 1997

Kevin turned over in bed, opened his eyes, and stared up at the ceiling. He focused only on the white expanse above. For a moment, it seemed as if the events of yesterday were a bad dream. His vision seemed to be just fine in this position.

Then he sat up.

His familiar surroundings were shrouded in an unfamiliar fog. A washed-out, colorless mist enveloped his room.

Grabbing the newspaper, he tried once again to read. No luck. The only satisfaction he got was from the full-page fashion ads, the ones that didn't need words, just glamorous pictures—Ralph Lauren, Tommy Hilfiger, Calvin Klein. Kevin enjoyed following the latest trends.

His frustration led him back to the liquor cabinet. By ten o'clock he was drinking vodka straight up.

He didn't bother with the colorless cranberry or orange juice. He knew vodka would dull the pain; its clean, comforting warmth had seen him through many trying times.

Kevin wondered how he'd managed to get through his high school years without it. He hadn't been as lucky in college.

* * *

Within the first few months of freshman year at Radford, a small liberal arts college in Radford, Virginia, Kevin started drinking during the fraternity rush period.

Kevin had his sights set on Pi Kappa Phi. He'd decided that was the cool frat, and he thought he had a chance to gain a bid.

He approached the impressive white, colonial house on Calhoun Street and stood out front gazing at it for a while. Finally, Kevin summoned the courage to walk onto the front porch.

He stood there, afraid to ring the doorbell.

He started to turn away when another prospective rush reached over Kevin's right shoulder and rang the bell. The door opened in an instant, as if someone had been waiting on the other side.

That someone was Skipper. He was wearing a smart navy-blue blazer that framed a loosely-knotted navy and burgundy striped tie. His trendy Vans were visible below his slightly too-short khakis. No socks, of course.

Kevin entered and was ushered to the basement where the keg served as the central form of entertainment for the night. Chip, the chief keg watchman, handed Kevin a beer in a sixteen-ounce blue plastic cup with the fraternity letters emblazoned in gold on it. He took a few gulps.

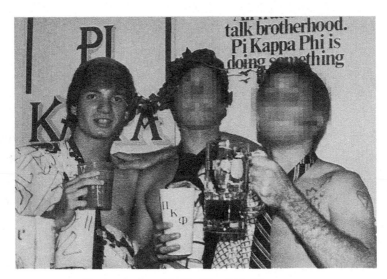

Kevin during his Radford College years

Chip shrugged his shoulders and offered the advice that would begin Kevin's descent into a lifelong battle against the bottle.

"Drink that down and grab a couple more. Then you'll be fine," he suggested casually.

Kevin downed the first cup and felt nothing. Halfway through the second cup, a warm feeling of contentment spread throughout his being.

Kevin liked it.

Aided by the good fortune of rarely getting sick or hung over, as well as the incentive to be the most respected pledge in his class, Kevin quickly graduated from being a non-drinker to someone who could consume nine thirty-ounce funnels of beer without too much trouble.

Kevin's love affair with liquid confidence had begun.

* * *

Kevin's eyesight had worsened considerably by Monday morning. Nevertheless, he was in the middle of a research project, and he knew his boss was waiting for the data. He made it a point to get to his office on thirty minutes earlier than normal.

After pouring his coffee, Kevin called a local ophthalmologist in his Murray Hill neighborhood. He lucked out and was given the first appointment the next day. He hoped this would be a quick visit, that he'd be fitted with a pair of glasses, and be back to work not long after his normal start time.

As Monday wore on, the simplicity of that scenario faded. Kevin found it increasingly difficult to read, and in turn, to concentrate. More than once that day he made up an excuse when his boss asked him about the status of the project.

The end of the workday couldn't come soon enough.

Kevin walked into his apartment that evening, threw his coat on the floor, and headed straight for the liquor cabinet. He poured himself a generous drink. He took several large gulps and topped it off. He turned and scanned his living room.

Kevin had style. He loved listening to music on his Bang and Olufsen stereo player. He owned a 1929 Corbusier-designed black leather sofa. Nelson benches on either side of his couch held exquisite art books—the Rothko, Mapplethorpe and Frankenthaler were three of his favorites. Gleaming silver frames displayed the photographs he'd taken over the years.

The drunker he got the more maudlin his thinking became. His fears became a reality in his alcohol-altered consciousness. He was never going to be able to see any of these treasured things again. He was sure of it in his gut, but he hid that knowledge even from himself. "I was just not going to go there," Kevin would later say.

* * *

Tuesday dawned bleak and bitter cold. Even the weather was against him. Kevin showered, got dressed, and headed the few blocks west to his eye doctor appointment.

There was no receptionist to greet him. He sat alone in the waiting area. Not being able to discern the words in the magazines he, nevertheless, flipped through the pages to pass the time. No sound came from behind the closed door to the ophthalmologist's examining room, and Kevin grew restless.

Had he misread the time on the clocks in his apartment? He just didn't know anymore.

After thirty minutes, the ophthalmologist, Dr. Michael, poked his head into the waiting room and motioned for Kevin to come on back. No apology was given and a rising anger added to Kevin's anxiety.

This was diffused a little when Kevin saw Dr. Michael's desk. It was an antique Biedermeier.

"Very striking desk," Kevin said.

"Yes, it is. I purchased it several years ago at an auction in Austria," Dr. Michael replied dismissively. "Now, tell me what's going on with your eyes."

Kevin didn't have the first sentence out before Dr. Michael's phone rang.

"Just a minute," he said, putting up one finger to indicate that he would only be a moment.

The minute became two, and then five, and then ten. Kevin started shifting in his seat. The voice on the other end of the line appeared to be Dr. Michael's stockbroker, and a protracted conversation about his portfolio of stocks and bonds was playing out. Dr. Michael didn't seem happy. Kevin shook his head in disbelief. The gesture caught Dr. Michael's attention, and he said his goodbyes.

"Sorry about that," Dr. Michael said. He wasn't sorry at all. "Now, where were we?"

Kevin started at the beginning relaying everything that had happened since the previous Thursday when he'd first noticed that he was unable to read. Dr. Michael appeared perplexed by the information and asked for clarification.

"*When* did you first notice you were having trouble reading?"

Kevin repeated his story. Still, Dr. Michael frowned as if he didn't understand. He asked Kevin to put his chin on the eye-examination machine chin rest. He adjusted the eyepieces and pulled up a low stool.

"Okay, I am going to start changing the lenses. Let me know which is clearer. Option one or option two."

Kevin tried hard to see a difference, but couldn't distinguish between either one. In fact, he couldn't see the letters very well at all.

"Neither option is clearer. I'm sorry, but I can't see a difference."

Kevin didn't understand why, but Dr. Michael seemed irritated. Biedermeier desk notwithstanding, Kevin was not liking this man's attitude at all.

Dr. Michael changed the lenses.

"Okay, how about these two choices, option A or option B?"

Kevin stared into the eyepieces again. He still couldn't see a difference. Dr. Michael flicked impatiently between option A and B asking in increasingly more urgent tones, "Option A or option B? Option A or option B?"

This was becoming a rapidly escalating nightmare. Kevin felt tears come to his eyes, further clouding his ability to distinguish between the choices.

"I'm sorry," he repeated. "I *can't* see any difference between the options you're showing me."

Dr. Michael pushed back from the machine and sighed.

"Are you being truthful with me? Some patients say what they think I want to hear. They don't want to admit they've got a problem even though they've come to see me about one."

Kevin was offended and found it difficult to form a reply.

"I'm not lying, Doctor Michael. I can't see any difference."

"Have you perhaps suffered from a traumatic experience within the last few days?"

"No," Kevin replied.

"Well, perhaps an injury? Or are you on drugs?"

"No, neither," Kevin answered firmly.

"Well, in my twenty-eight years of practice, I've never had a patient who's claimed to have such a sudden and dramatic sight loss."

The tears were now gone, and an irritation to match the doctor's was coming to the surface. Kevin pushed back his chair. Dr. Michael stood up from his stool.

"Make another appointment for next week," Dr. Michael suggested. "I'll be happy to retest you when you're in a better emotional state."

Kevin couldn't believe what he was hearing.

"I need some help today. Some glasses or something."

"I can't give you glasses if I don't know what's going on with you. Make another appointment for next week."

With that, Kevin was dismissed from the examining room. The receptionist was now at her desk, but Kevin wouldn't be making another appointment. He pulled out his checkbook to pay the first and final bill. The tears came back. He couldn't see well enough to fill out the check. He swallowed his pride and asked her for help.

Kevin didn't try to make it to his office. He returned home and poured himself a stiff one. The first gulps steadied his nerves. He called in sick and then telephoned his mother.

"Mom, I made the eye appointment like you asked, but the doctor wasn't able to help me. Can you please ask your doctor for a referral?"

"I'll call you back in a few hours," Ruth promised. Kevin couldn't help noticing the edge in her voice. He knew he had alarmed his mother and felt guilty about having to ask her for help.

When Ruth called back two hours later, Kevin was on his third tumbler of straight-up vodka. His mother sounded hopeful, and Kevin's spirits lifted for a brief moment.

"Okay, Kevin, I have two names for you. Both are neuro-ophthalmologists, and both are experts in their field."

Kevin called the first doctor and was told there was a two-month wait for the first open appointment. He decided to put a bit more urgency into his request when he called the second person his mother had given him—a Dr. Myles from Columbia Presbyterian Medical Center.

"Hello, this is an emergency," he said, as soon as the receptionist answered the phone. "I've lost almost all of my vision within the last three days; I'm thirty-six years old and otherwise healthy. My name is Kevin Coughlin."

He was given the first appointment Thursday morning.

SELECTED JOURNAL ENTRY:

February 21, 2014—the fog I'm seeing this morning is environmental rather than the dense, milky fog that has been my ever-present reality.

CHAPTER 3

Dart Boards

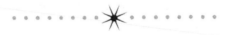

Thursday, February 20, 1997

Kevin was clinging to a fragile hope. He vacillated between accepting his reality and evading the fact he was losing his sight. The booze, which had become his foe, was at this point his unintended friend, enabling him to numb his emotions.

Entering the doctor's office, he took in his surroundings, recording things as if to store them away in his mind's eye for future reference. The day might come when that would be the last place he could see things.

He could still see large objects, such as chairs, but he could no longer distinguish their color. Likewise, he could see the outline of the paintings that lined the walls, but he had no idea whether they were landscapes or abstracts—they were just a blur of muted shades of gray. A round table of some type of dark wood displayed magazines. He didn't bother picking one up.

He was nervous, but today, at least, he wasn't kept waiting in anxiety. Dr. Myles appeared in the doorway of the waiting room within moments of Kevin's arrival. Kevin couldn't see him clearly, but his voice alone painted a portrait of compassion and competence. Kevin could see well enough to tell that he was tall and carried himself in a stately manner.

"Come on back," Dr. Myles said, extending his right arm until his hand touched Kevin's. Kevin smiled, realizing Dr. Myles was making sure Kevin could see he wanted to shake his hand.

"Has anyone ever mentioned that you're the spitting image of that British actor Michael York?" Dr. Myles said.

Many people had asked Kevin this same question. Normally he would put on an actor's pose in response, raising an arched eyebrow, but he wasn't able to offer more than a weak smile in reply to Dr. Myles.

He followed Dr. Myles into the small examination room. Kevin was holding his head to the left—an indication he was trying hard to focus out of what remained of his left peripheral vision. He could see Dr. Myles looking intently at him, as if he was making mental notes even before he started to make written ones.

"Why don't we start at the beginning, Kevin," Dr. Myles suggested. "Tell me when you first noticed that you had trouble with your vision."

Kevin couldn't speak. He knew where to begin but couldn't.

"Take your time. Just tell me what's been going on," Dr. Myles said calmly. The tears that seemed to be coming with easy frequency over the last several days welled up again. Kevin fought for control.

"On Saturday, I couldn't read the newspaper. Later that day I visited my parents, and I couldn't read my mother's grocery list or see the color of my mother's eyes—they're a vibrant blue."

Kevin put his forefingers to the corners of his eyes to dab away his tears, embarrassed by them. Dr. Myles didn't seem to notice; he was busy taking notes.

"Okay, let's start with a basic old-fashioned test," he suggested, motioning for Kevin to follow him to the other side of the examining room. "I've got lots of newfangled machinery, but I find this simple test is a good place to start. It will evaluate your central vision."

Kevin trusted Dr. Myles. Such a difference between this appointment and the one he had on Tuesday!

Kevin sat down in front of a grid-like screen that resembled an oversized dart board—circles within circles with degrees plotted on them. Dr. Myles explained what was about to happen.

"I'm going to hold up three different colored socks, one at a time. Blue, red, and yellow. Look straight ahead at the board. As I move these socks in front of your face, please let me know when they first appear."

Dr. Myles held up the first sock and slowly moved it, left to right, in front of Kevin's face. Nothing appeared in Kevin's right periphery or central vision. Dr. Myles did the same exercise with the next sock, and finally, the third. Kevin was only able to see the socks from the far edge of his left peripheral vision. The test took a long time. Two hours.

"Can you come back tomorrow for another test?" Dr. Myles asked.

Kevin registered Dr. Myles' concern.

"What do you think is wrong?"

"I have a hunch, but I'd rather wait for further test results." Once again, Kevin's tears welled up. Kevin pushed for reassurance.

"Can you fix it? Are there any treatments?"

Dr. Myles repeated that he wanted to wait for the second round of test results. They stood up and shook hands. "Kevin, if you smoke or drink, please stop immediately."

Kevin didn't smoke, and he had no intention to stop drinking. He didn't bother asking Dr. Myles for an explanation. Many years later, he would wish that he had.

Kevin left the office and headed to one of his favorite bars, The Oscar Wilde, on 58th Street between First and Second Avenues. The Oscar Wilde was the typical New York City dark mahogany bar—not fancy, although not a dive either.

Kevin had a fleeting irrational moment of concern that Dr. Myles might catch him there, yet he couldn't imagine that this would be the type of place Dr. Myles frequented. It would have been safer altogether to drink at his apartment, but right now Kevin wanted the comfort of other people. Not only that, he wanted to pretend that his world wasn't falling apart. He'd have a drink in a bar, maybe two, just like anyone else.

His charade lasted until he needed to use the restroom. He thought he knew the bar well enough to navigate his way there. However, as he walked away from the brightness of the bar itself, the darkness of the corridors overwhelmed him.

He thought he had found the men's room and was now desperate to relieve himself when he heard someone rustling around.

He was in the cloak room!

Readjusting his trousers, he stumbled back into the bar. Between the drinks he had consumed and his impaired vision, it was hard not to bump into tables, chairs, and people on the way out. He knocked over someone's drink.

"Hey, watch where you're going. You just spilled my drink."

Kevin reached into his pocket and threw some bills down on the bar. He headed out into daylight, but his descent into darkness had officially begun.

SELECTED JOURNAL ENTRY:

March 1, 2014—for the entire duration of the blindness, I felt tightness in my neck and upper back. I just accepted it, as I attributed it to the stress of dealing with navigating the world without sight. But I am now having a realization—the long-held stiffness is mysteriously subsiding.

CHAPTER 4

Dashed Hopes

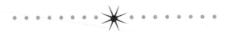

Friday, February 21-Sunday, February 23, 1997

Kevin slept fitfully. He was almost glad when his alarm clock went off Friday morning. He made his way to the bathroom, tilting his head to the side to gain as much access to his remaining peripheral vision as possible. Nevertheless, he bumped into his couch along the way.

He dressed and ate breakfast quickly. He headed out to Lexington Avenue to hail a cab. Despite the bitter February temperatures, and hence a dearth of cabs, one stopped for him within a few minutes. Kevin thought this might be a good sign. He headed back up to Dr. Myles' office.

Friday was a long day. Kevin endured a battery of demoralizing tests, one of which was to rule out inoperable brain cancer. At this point, Kevin was not sure this would have been bad news. The doctors also checked his blood for diabetes and various forms of vitamin deficiencies. The worst tests, however, were the series of MRI's. The incessant banging in the machine eerily matched the banging in Kevin's head.

* * *

Kevin stayed in his apartment all day on Saturday and waited for Dr. Myles to call. He'd promised Kevin that he would phone by Sunday morning at the latest. Kevin was holding on to the thinnest of hopes that everything would be okay despite his worsening eyesight.

When the phone rang on Sunday morning, Kevin nearly tripped over his coffee table as he dashed to answer it. Even the phone's ring sounded ominous.

"Kevin, this is Dr. Myles. I've looked over all the tests. The good news is that you don't have a brain tumor. The bad news is that I am now all but certain that you have a genetic disorder called Leber's Hereditary Optic Neuropathy. The only thing giving me some pause is that Leber's normally affects people in their teens or early twenties, and the sight deterioration is generally over weeks, or even months, not days. Although it does primarily affect men."

Kevin's head started to pound. The *on the one hand this, and on the other hand that* discourse started to fade into the distance. He grabbed his ears and slid to the floor. As soon as his head cleared, he started firing questions at Dr. Myles.

"Are there any drugs? An operation? Is there any hope for me?"

Dr. Myles was silent for a few moments. "Can you come back next Thursday? Before I try to answer your questions, I'd like to run some more tests."

More tests!

Kevin tried to pour a vodka without making any obvious clinking sounds with his glass. He turned away from the phone and took a gulp. He closed his eyes and swallowed hard.

"What tests?" he asked.

"I'd like to schedule an appointment for you with a neuro-geneticist to do a DNA test."

"Dr. Myles, is my sight going to come back or not?" Kevin asked bluntly. The vodka was already working.

"Kevin, I know this is hard. We have to wait until we get the test results back. And a DNA test takes time. It could be June before we get the final results."

"June—that's four months from now!" exclaimed Kevin. "Isn't there anything I can do that will help me now?" The doctor's pause increased Kevin's mounting fear.

"The only thing some people believe might slow down the progression of sight loss is extreme amounts of vitamins—L-carnitine, coenzyme Q10 and a B-complex."

"I'll buy them right away," Kevin said, "but that's just slowing down the loss, right? Isn't there anything I can do to help restore my lost vision?" There was another moment of silence that seemed to drag on for hours.

"Let's wait until we get the test results back," Dr. Myles repeated.

Kevin's heart sank. He tried to console himself with the fact that he did have some of his left peripheral vision. "Well, worst case scenario, I can still see a bit from my left side. I'll get to keep that, right?"

In the ensuing silence, Kevin heard the answer.

SELECTED JOURNAL ENTRY:

April 14, 2014—today is the first day that my vision appears to be worse. It is gray, blurry, and exceedingly pixilated. However, I feel with every ounce of my being, every cell that something incredible is stirring. My optic nerve is undergoing a gut renovation—a rebirth!

CHAPTER 5

ABV

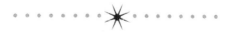

Monday, February 24, 1997

Kevin woke up Monday morning with a raging hangover. He didn't bother to try to make it to work or even call in sick. He knew he would lose his job, and by the end of the week, he had. At least, he was able to apply for social security disability and food stamps. He didn't blame his employer—a blind man could hardly do marketing research.

Kevin called his friend Rob and asked him to google Leber's. The first hit was on the National Institute of Health's website.

"It's sort of long and complicated," he told Kevin. "Should I just read it to you?"

"Sure," Kevin replied reluctantly. He wasn't at all sure he was ready to hear more bad news, especially so early on Monday morning before he'd had a drink. Rob began to read.

"Leber's Hereditary Optic Neuropathy (LHON) is an inherited form of sight loss. Theodor Leber was a German ophthalmologist who first described the disease in 1871. Although this condition generally begins in a person's teens or twenties, rare cases can occur in early childhood or in later adulthood. For unknown reasons, males are affected much more often than females. Blurring and clouding of vision are usually the first symptoms of this disorder. These vision problems may begin in one eye or appear simultaneously in both eyes; if vision loss starts in one eye, it usually occurs in the other within several weeks or months. Over time, vision loss worsens in both eyes, resulting in a severe loss of sharpness (visual acuity) as well as color vision."

"This condition produces loss of central vision, which is needed for detailed tasks, such as driving, reading and recognizing faces. Vision loss results from the death of cells in the optic nerve that relays information from the eyes to the brain. Although central vision gradually improves in a small percentage of cases, in most cases the vision loss is profound and permanent."

Kevin's head started to spin again. The words "profound and permanent" had the effect of eliminating the last bit of hope Kevin held.

By the time Kevin had finished his conversation with Dr. Myles the night before, he'd emptied his vodka reserves and was in need of a refill.

Urgent need.

Kevin's drinking had progressed in the last twenty years to the point of alcoholism. What had started out as too many beers in the frat house basement had escalated to too many drinks on the weekends, and eventually, to too many straight-up vodkas every day.

As soon as it turned 10 a.m., Kevin set out for the closest liquor store. Wood Spirits was only one block away. Nevertheless, Kevin knew the short trip would not be easy. Wood was an impressive establishment. With its mahogany veneers, crystal decanters, and daily wine tastings, it was not any ordinary liquor store. Wood billed itself as a purveyor of fine spirits.

Kevin didn't need any top-shelf brands that morning. He needed ABV—alcohol by volume. He would get a handle. Any half-gallon jug would do. Kevin was now not only thinking like an alcoholic, he *was* one.

Kevin crossed Lexington Avenue and found himself at the top of Murray Hill. He proceeded with caution, hugging the right side of the jagged building line. After several yards, he was gratified when he touched the gate of an apartment building on his right-hand side. He'd always admired this distinctive gate and now knew where he was.

He groped his way—a man in the dark. At midblock, he swept his hands across the low flung black iron gate of another brownstone, again to determine his bearings. At the same moment, a woman's voice shouted out from a window above.

"Hey, what do you want?"

Kevin looked up in the direction of the voice even though he knew he would not be able to see the woman. He must have appeared disheveled.

"Are you on drugs?" she cried. "Please...get out of here or I'm calling the police." Kevin was dumbstruck. Had he really fallen that low?

Being mistaken for a drug addict stumbling around Murray Hill had riled Kevin up. His dignity needed to be restored, and he knew he was the only one that could do it. As he walked back to his apartment from Wood, Kevin formulated a plan. He wasted no time putting it into action.

Kevin held no reservations whatsoever concerning psychotherapy, having previously experienced its benefits. He had spent six years in therapy in his twenties coming to terms with his sexuality.

It had not been easy for Kevin to accept that he was gay. A good Catholic boy was expected to marry a good Catholic girl and produce good Catholic children. Kevin had tried to comply. He even had a girlfriend, Elyse, for three years at Radford. But by the time he'd graduated, he'd "confessed" the truth to her, as well as, to himself.

Kevin held no illusions about the commitment of time and emotional energy that therapy required. He decided he would find a support group before seeking individual counseling. Although he'd never been to one, nor had knowledge of how they functioned, he believed in the adage that there was strength in numbers.

His first call was to a renowned New York City agency dedicated to serving the blind and visually impaired.

"Hello, I'm calling to inquire about your services for the blind," Kevin began.

"The intake person is on vacation for two weeks, but I'll connect you to her voice mail," replied the receptionist, as if reading from a script.

"Just a minute please," Kevin said attempting to interrupt her to say that his call was rather urgent. It was too late—the receptionist had hung up, and Kevin was connected to the intake woman's voice mail. Undaunted, he called again.

"Hello, I understand that the normal intake person is on vacation for two weeks, but would you please connect me to someone else in the intake department who is currently available to make an appointment?" Kevin didn't let her get away this time. "I have suddenly lost almost all of my vision, and I need to speak to someone right away."

This seemed to get her attention, but it didn't get the result Kevin wanted.

"Sir, the records indicate that the first available appointment for a low-vision evaluation would be in ten weeks' time."

Kevin was still undaunted.

"Okay, thanks, before you hang up the phone, could you please connect me with someone who has knowledge of support groups?" The receptionist transferred Kevin's call.

The new voice identified herself as a social worker and asked how she could be of assistance. Kevin gave her a short description of his sight loss and explained that he was in urgent need of locating a support group.

"I'm afraid that none of our support groups would fit your needs," she replied. Puzzled, Kevin asked her to explain.

"The vast majority of people who experience vision loss are senior citizens who slowly lose their sight as a result of conditions such as glaucoma or macular degeneration. Our other support group services teenagers who are blind from birth and just need a little help navigating their blindness during the tricky period of adolescence."

"There must be some group that can help people like me," Kevin interjected. The social worker sighed signaling the fact that there was nothing else she could do; she nevertheless continued to explain the predicament further.

"Blindness is a low-incidence disability affecting less than one percent of the population. And it is extremely rare for someone at your age to experience such significant and rapid vision loss."

Kevin had heard this same thing from Dr. Myles, but that didn't soften the blow.

"Well, is there any group that can help people like me?" Kevin asked again in a last-ditch effort.

"You could try the Jewish Guild for the Blind," the social worker offered. "They might be able to help."

Kevin was too frustrated to make any more calls that day and opted instead for several stiff drinks, even though he knew the anesthetizing effect would be temporary. By the time Kevin stumbled into bed that night, he knew he needed more help than a liquor bottle, full or empty, could provide.

SELECTED JOURNAL ENTRY:

May 10, 2014—I now consistently have depth of field, and I'm beginning to see weather conditions as they actually are.

CHAPTER 6

Seeking Support

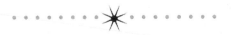

Tuesday, February 25-Thursday, February 27, 1997

On Tuesday morning Kevin summoned the energy to call the Jewish Guild. The receptionist was a delight—a complete contrast to his previous day's experience. Where there had been cold indifference, there was kindness and compassion.

"Good morning, my name is Gloria, how can I assist you?' she said with such warmth that Kevin was immediately at ease.

Kevin repeated his story. Gloria was quick to help.

"Do you have a few minutes to complete an intake questionnaire over the phone?"

Kevin's spirits lifted. An intake—right then over the phone. No ten-week wait for an appointment!

The first set of questions were routine—name and address, age, eye condition. She then explained the required paperwork—certification of legal blindness from the state of New York and registration with the New York State Commission for the Blind and Visually Handicapped.

Being classified as handicapped did not sit well with Kevin. It invoked an image of damaged or broken goods, however, Gloria was being nice and Kevin brushed it off. After the initial intake was completed, Gloria transferred Kevin to a social worker who had more familiarity with support groups.

Again, Kevin was delighted to be connected with someone who evoked patience and kindness, even though he proceeded to repeat almost verbatim what the previous social worker had said about the dearth of appropriate support groups. There was one significant difference—a new suggestion.

"There is another group. It's a long shot, but it might be worth looking into."

"I'll try anything."

"Well, Kevin, the group I have in mind is at the Gay Men's Health Crisis. It's for individuals who have experienced sudden vision loss or blindness such as yourself, however, as a result of HIV-related infections or conditions. There might be one problem though—the group is limited to individuals who are HIV positive and are clients of GMHC. That said, if you're game, let's give it a shot."

Although Kevin was HIV negative, he had more than a passing acquaintance with GMHC having volunteered there as a Buddy for men with AIDS for over three years. He thought this fact would increase his chances of being accepted into the support group.

Kevin called the GMHC and was connected to Mark, the group facilitator, who began by explaining the logistics and ended by asking the all-important question.

"Are you a client of the agency?" Kevin was quick to reply, explaining his mitigating circumstances.

"No, but I have been a Buddy for three years and really need this group."

"Look, Kevin, I feel empathy for you, but I don't make the rules. The group is off limits to non-clients. I'm really very sorry. I truly am."

As Kevin had such high hopes, he was devastated. He kept Mark on the line, pouring himself a serious vodka while balancing the phone to his ear. He would once again numb the harsh reality he had just been dealt.

"Isn't there someone else I can speak to about my request? Perhaps your supervisor?"

"I'm really sorry," repeated Mark.

* * *

Kevin was not about to give up. The next morning, he placed another call to the GMHC. This time, he was connected with Mary Ann, a graduate school intern who was the co-facilitator of the group. Kevin felt Mary Ann's compassion. She was young and idealistic, and she explained to Kevin that she was prepared to go to battle for him.

"I'll speak with Mark," she promised. "I'll plead your case." For a moment, Kevin thought she might be a skilled trial attorney. "I'll call you back when I have news," she promised.

Mary Ann proved good to her word. When she called to tell Kevin that she had convinced Mark to discuss Kevin's possible participation with the group, and that the group *had* agreed to accept him, she was bubbling over with excitement. She relayed the common position of the group by repeating what one member had said.

"Our group is about learning to deal with loss of vision—not managing our HIV status. So, let's give him our support!"

This was Kevin's first victory in a long, drawn out, brutal battle. Not only was he confronting the crushing loss of sight, he had to deal with bureaucracy, poverty, depression, red tape, and institutionalized indifference along the way.

However, each conflict and bureaucratic hurdle also served to make Kevin stronger and more assertive. The blindness made him feel invisible. He was determined to remedy that by having a voice.

* * *

Kevin's first session with the visually impaired support group on Wednesday morning was extraordinary on many levels.

The group members introduced themselves. There was Edgar, who had cytomegalovirus (CMV). He had gone to sleep one night with perfect vision and woke up the next morning blind. Bill also had CMV, as well as cataracts.

Al, the Peter-Pan of the group, introduced himself as an aging club kid who loved the nightlife. He had severe cataracts and tended to wear sunglasses even indoors. David admitted that he had the best vision of anyone in the group. He had had a partially detached retina as well as a cataract, but both conditions had been corrected with surgery. He attended the group as a precautionary measure to emotionally prepare himself in the event he might lose more of his vision.

Pablo was the comedian and described himself as buff and just as hot as Edgar. He was blind, having lost his vision the previous year from meningitis. The two newest members of the group were Ken and Sunshine. Ken suffered from CMV, and Sunshine, the group's only female member, whose positive attitude and spirit bore witness to her moniker, had lost her vision as a result of meningitis, as well. After the introductions, Kevin told his story. Never before had he felt so much love and acceptance; never before had he allowed himself to be so open and vulnerable. It felt so freeing—like a thousand-pound weight had been lifted from his shoulders.

Kevin returned to his apartment after the meeting drained and exhausted. But, he only had two stiff drinks that night instead of his customary three or four.

SELECTED JOURNAL ENTRY:

June 22, 2014—as I am waiting in front of my building, I see water flowing from a hose. Omar is watering the plants.

CHAPTER 7

Blind Man's Bluff

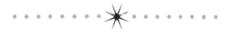

Spring 1997

In those first critical months of Kevin's blindness the group was invaluable to him. It was his lifeline, his sustenance. He soon learned from his fellow members that blindness was not a death sentence.

In addition to providing Kevin with inspiration and motivation, the group also offered him practical advice and guidance. For example, Pablo taught Kevin how to organize the money in his wallet. His billfold was divided into two sections. The ones went in the first section, followed by the fives, folded in half. Then the tens in the second section, followed by twenties, again folded in half.

When Kevin complained about the difficulty of switching his razor blades, the group suggested using disposable blades or an electric one instead. He also learned how to listen for traffic patterns so he knew when it was safe to cross the street, and to organize his CD collection into alphabetical rows so he could locate his favorite songs.

Most important of all was the companionship of the group. Friday evening get-togethers would begin in Bill's ultra-chic digs in Chelsea.

Some weeks it was just Bill and Kevin. Other times the guest list would include Ken and Sunshine, or Pablo and his partner. After happy hour in Bill's loft, they would order Chinese food or venture out for dinner to a neighborhood restaurant.

They'd often laugh in the face of adversity, finding humor in tragic or absurd situations. One day, Sunshine exclaimed that she was wearing a beautiful floral print scarf, explaining that even though she had never been very girly, she could now wear her mother's collection of beaded necklaces and silk scarves without seeing how garish they looked on her. She then somehow transitioned with ease to how two days earlier she had a port installed in her neck to simplify her daily medication infusions.

On another occasion, Ken shrieked that he hated going out with his pathetic white cane. His solution was to cover it with a tasteful black and white houndstooth print of cotton fabric.

"If I have to be blind, at least I can do it with a little style!"

There was no pretense, no judgment—just unbridled acceptance. Kevin began to feel safe.

Despite all the benefits of the group, Kevin started to feel guilty that all he had to deal with was blindness, while the others were also fighting for their lives. One day he expressed his reservations about staying in the group. Ken put him in his place.

"Get over it, Kevin! It's not a cold that you caught. You've lost your vision for God's sake. That is enough. You belong here."

And so Kevin stayed. He now felt truly connected and accepted, not an outsider. Best of all, he was no longer alone in his dark, unfamiliar world.

The support group boosted Kevin's morale, and he was now able to face some indisputable truths with a new confidence. It wasn't long before he accepted the fact that he would need the universal symbol that told the world he was blind.

A white cane.

As he set out to buy his first one, he smiled again at Ken's announcement that he had a customized black and white hounds-tooth model. How would Kevin decorate his?

The authorized store that sold canes was located in the lobby of an agency serving the blind. Kevin hoped buying a cane would be a better experience than his initial run-in with this agency in February.

Although by this point Kevin had mastered buying clothes, a cane was not exactly an item he'd any experience shopping for yet. It was another first of the many that had so rudely interrupted his life.

Upon his arrival at the agency, the store manager, greeted him.

"Good morning, I'm Henry, how can I help you?"

"I'd like to buy a cane," Kevin said.

"Hmm, you look about six feet tall," Henry said, assessing the exact cane size to fit Kevin's height. "The tip of the handle should fall between the sternum and pectoral area of the chest," he explained. The fifty-four-inch model did just that. With the appropriate cane size determined, Kevin assumed the next logical thing was to simply pay for it. He offered Henry his credit card.

"Are you certified as being mobile?" Henry asked.

Kevin paused at Henry's question. He had never heard that someone had to be certified as mobile before being allowed to buy a cane. His warning antennae went up; nevertheless, he answered truthfully.

"No, I haven't taken mobility training yet. I'm on the waiting list, and I will begin in four months."

Henry spoke somewhat apologetically but it didn't soften the blow.

"I'm sorry, sir. In that case, I can't sell you the cane today."

"What do you mean?"

"Store policy only allows me to sell canes to patrons who have completed mobility training and are certified by New York State as being safe and mobile."

Yet another brick wall.

Kevin's normal polite manner started to crack. He asked the next obvious question.

"So…what am I to do in the meantime?"

"I understand your predicament, sir. While I don't make the rules, I'm nevertheless obligated to make sure they are followed. And I'll certainly be here to help when you're certified." With that, and before Kevin could register a further complaint, he heard Henry walk toward the other side of the store.

His confidence and good humor gone, Kevin turned to leave. Just as he reached the door, someone walked in. Henry's voice rang out almost instantly in her direction.

"Good morning, young lady. How may I help you?"

"I'm an actress, and I'm doing research for an upcoming role as a blind person. I want to understand about canes and how to use them."

"And naturally, you want your performance to be authentic," said Henry understandingly.

Kevin paused by the exit, lingering within eavesdropping distance.

"Could you show me how to grip the handle please?" The young actress asked in a sweet, almost child-like, tone.

To his astonishment, Kevin heard a two-minute mobility lesson. Henry explained that there was a rhythm to using a cane that was similar to ballroom dancing.

"Hold the cane in the center of your body. First, tap the cane on the surface of the ground from left to right. Before you take a step with your left foot, the cane should be in front of your left foot, and likewise, before you step with your right foot."

Then the actress in her came to the fore as she spoke even more sweetly to Henry and asked, "I don't suppose I could…"

"Borrow the cane to study for your part? Of course! Just be sure to please return it when you're done. Let me get some contact information from you," Henry replied with such enthusiasm that Kevin almost lost his temper.

Kevin could not believe what he had heard. An actress in need of a prop to prepare for a role was going to be provided with a cane, free of charge, while he, a man who had just gone blind and in urgent need, was denied the right to even purchase one. Incensed by the insanity of this, he joined the conversation and confronted Henry.

"Are you really going to lend a cane to this actress, and refuse to sell one to someone who is truly in need?"

The startled actress wasn't acting now.

"Wait! You're going to lend me a cane to rehearse for a TV show, but you're denying this man one? Someone who obviously truly needs it?"

Henry had no reasonable reply. As manager of the store, he had to enforce the rules. However, as he had demonstrated with the actress, he could also bend them. A combination of the young woman's incredulity combined with Kevin's persistence produced the intended result—Kevin left the store with a graphite white cane in hand, as well as, a two-minute mobility lesson on how to use it.

A compassionate actress, all the makings of a television drama, and a happy ending had occurred. Buoyed by a restored confidence—and his newfound cane—Kevin tapped his way out of the store. He thought he had just mastered the most challenging part of his new, dark world.

His assumption, like so many others, soon proved ill-founded.

SELECTED JOURNAL ENTRY:

July 21, 2014—patience, prayer, and turmeric; the foundation, the corner stones of my journey out of the darkness.

CHAPTER 8

Shattered Beauty

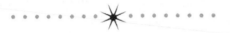

Summer 1997

As the summer temperatures started to climb, and what was left of his peripheral vision deteriorated, Kevin found his hopes dwindling. He'd tried to broach the subject of his eyesight with his parents several times, but they were too upset to discuss it.

In June, the last thin thread broke when he received the definitive conclusions of the genetic test. He had indeed inherited the LHON gene from his mother.

Kevin would never see again.

He'd been drinking throughout the day. By the time the news came, he was quite drunk. Alcohol was no longer just the friend that dulled his emotions. Now it also fueled his anger.

He flew into a rage.

What the hell was the use of all the beautiful things in his apartment? If he was never going to see them again, then he didn't want them around. He began to systematically destroy everything that he loved. The first things to go were his own prized photographs.

Thrown. Shattered. Stepped and stomped upon.

Kevin was quite a good amateur photographer which made his sudden blindness both a physical handicap, as well as, a loss of his creative outlet.

He hurled his Swedish crystal bowls at the walls and yanked his prized paintings off their hooks. Kevin stepped on some shattered glass and cut his foot. A fair amount of his blood spotted the living room floor along with the debris caused by his own destruction.

Then as abruptly as Kevin had started destroying things, he stopped.

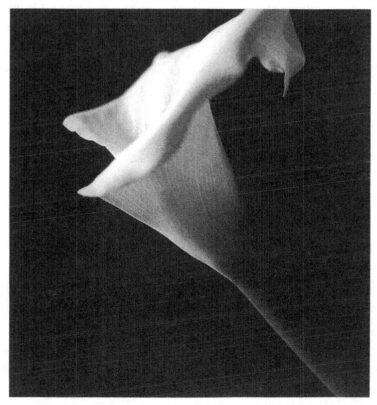

"Calla Lily" by Kevin Coughlin

Music. Music would calm him. He stepped over the debris and stood in front of his beloved Bang & Olufsen stereo. He ran his hands over the sleek, brushed aluminum and smoked glass. He decided to play his favorite songs, sit down with another drink, and clean up the mess later.

The intended calm didn't come. Unable to find the electronic green arrow that controlled the opening and closing of the CD player, Kevin became agitated again. He began pushing here and there on the smooth control panel in the hope of hitting the right button by chance. The CD player stayed resolutely shut.

Kevin gripped the sides of the stereo player and hoisted it from the table, yanking the wires from the speakers and the electric cords from the wall. He stepped out into the hallway of his apartment building and tossed it with all his might down the trash chute. He then fell back against the wall, panting, as if he'd just run five miles.

Then he smiled.

Who would find it? Who would be treated to a high-end, state-of-the-art Bang & Olufsen the next morning?

* * *

By the end of the summer, Kevin decided that he couldn't put off telling his parents the bad news any longer. While he had shared Dr. Myles' preliminary diagnosis with them in February, they had held on to the fragile belief that something could be done to restore Kevin's eyesight.

It was Friday of Labor Day weekend. Kevin had wanted to lay low in the city. It had been several months since he'd seen his parents, and he decided to surprise them. He set off for their house on Long Island—a trip that had once been routine had now become an act of courage, perseverance, and luck. Traversing the crowded platforms of Penn

Station required more than Kevin's determination due to the massive number of New Yorkers heading out to the Long Island beaches for the holiday.

His mother was home alone when he arrived. He found her at the kitchen table, dragging on a cigarette and clicking her tongue as she read the newspaper. Princess Diana had been killed in a car crash in Paris the night before. Kevin was glad his father wasn't there. The news would be marginally easier to deliver to his mother alone.

"Mom, could you come and sit with me in the living room, please? There's something I need to tell you." She looked up from the newspaper for the first time. She put her cigarette out and wiped her eyes.

"What's wrong?" she asked.

"Come in to the living room. Please."

Kevin couldn't see the anxiety on his mother's face. If he had been able to, he would have seen the transition from sadness over Princess Diana's death to concern over what her son was about to tell her.

"Mom," Kevin began haltingly, "the genetic test results arrived." Silence. "They confirmed that I do have Leber's, and I will never see again. My eyesight is not coming back."

Kevin paused to allow his mother to process the information. He was used to his parents' discomfort in talking about his blindness. Even though it was irrational, they both blamed themselves for having "given" Kevin the gene that led to it. Kevin braced himself for his mother's response.

"Did you know that your sister and Tom bought a business in Saratoga? They're planning on building a house there."

Even against the backdrop of his parents' avoidance, Kevin was shocked. For a moment, he thought that his mother must not have heard him.

"Mom, did you hear what I just said?"

Her second reply was even more of a non-sequitur.

"You really loved Princess Diana too, didn't you?"

Realizing this was his mother's way of coping with his news, of absorbing the tragic by invoking the mundane, Kevin simply replied, "Yes, mom, I did."

His father offered Kevin the most support that weekend. As a result of his stroke, Walter needed extra assistance performing daily tasks. Kevin helped him to bed that night. As Kevin was about to turn out his father's reading light, he touched Kevin's arm.

"Mom always said that the worst thing that ever happened to our family was my stroke," his father said. "But she was wrong. The worst thing to ever happen to our family is your blindness; I'm so sorry about your news."

Kevin started to choke up. Before he could respond, his father continued.

"You are doing so well, and I am so proud of you. I know you are going to be fine."

Despite his mother's non-response to the genetic test results, Kevin's father's love and unexpected encouragement bolstered his courage. Once again, Kevin felt he could forge ahead with renewed confidence.

SELECTED JOURNAL ENTRY:

August 22, 2014—when I wake up in the middle of the night, my vision is like looking directly through the ocean as waves gently roll in. It is not blue like the ocean but punctuated by various shades of gray.

CHAPTER 9

Finding Faith

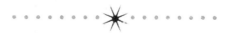

Fall 1997

Fall arrived with good news.

Kevin learned that he was, at long last, eligible to begin individual counseling at the Jewish Guild for the Blind. Since he was still not yet technically "certified mobile" despite the clever procurement of a cane with the help of the willing actress, he didn't push his luck. He took a car service to the Guild for his weekly therapy session.

Kevin had a good feeling about his therapist, Faith, from the start. Kevin always appreciated it when people he met for the first time offered a physical description of themselves so that he could "see" them. Despite her warmth, Faith shared only that she had brown hair and was wearing an engagement ring. Kevin wanted to know more, of course, yet decided not to push the issue during their first visit.

His first session with Faith was an instant success. Kevin experienced a profound sense of relief even before it was over. Although the GMHC group continued to be therapeutic for him, there were some things that he didn't feel comfortable sharing in that forum. Kevin continued to believe that the life and death issues the other group members confronted on a daily basis dwarfed his sudden vision loss, even though the impact of it was huge for him.

Blind though he was, he was also very much alive.

His sessions with Faith offered him a venue to express his sadness about his loss without feeling self-conscious about it. He was able to voice the pain of no longer being able to see the spire of the Chrysler Building as he entered his apartment. Or seeing the way his beloved dog, a Weimaraner named Pepper, danced with excitement when he returned home. Or simply to see his favorite visual images—the ocean, skyscrapers, and white flowers.

Faith was instrumental in helping Kevin understand that he too had experienced a type of death. His sight had been a vital, living, breathing part of his life that had been stripped away with no warning.

"Sudden blindness is very hard on anyone," Faith said. "But you were such a visual person, an amateur photographer and designer. You need to give yourself time and permission to grieve your loss." Kevin knew Faith was right. He began to allow himself to experience and mourn his loss. Even though most of his sessions with Faith were pleasant and constructive, they couldn't find a common ground over the issue of his cane.

"What I hate about using the cane is that I am now definitively BLIND! People on the street will see me as pathetic." Faith was sympathetic but pulled no punches.

"Unfortunately, Kevin, there is no getting around the fact that you are blind. After all, isn't that why you're here? In terms of labels, however, no one is putting a label of pathetic on you. Only you can do that to yourself." Kevin ignored her valid point and continued to complain.

"What I really don't like is that the cane is right in your face. It screams out 'blind guy on board!' Maybe I should wrap it in houndstooth cloth like Ken did. I actually did wonder how I should decorate it." Faith was not convinced.

"I wouldn't recommend decorating in any way at all, Kevin. The cane is white and distinctive for your safety. It lets people know that you're blind, and they need to use extra care when passing you on the street." Kevin acknowledged Faith's explanation, and then delved into the underlying issue.

"What's so difficult, what the real issue is, is that the cane is another dreadful reminder that I am not in the driver's seat. There is so little in my life that I can control anymore."

Kevin was an intelligent man. Faith tried a more philosophical approach.

"I'm sure you've heard this before, Kevin, but control is merely an illusion. None of us is ever really in control." Kevin sat up and smiled in agreement. Faith finished her thought.

"Perhaps you can flip this all on its side by changing your perspective. Sometimes you have to give up control to get it." Kevin knew Faith's advice was sound, and he vowed right then and there to attempt to follow it.

SELECTED JOURNAL ENTRY:

September 13, 2014—my view of the external environment is changing from one of black, white, and gray to multiple shades of beige.

CHAPTER 10

Brave New World

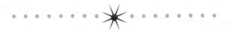

Winter 1998

Still untrained, and therefore, self-conscious, Kevin used his cane only when he walked Pepper. The more he tried to use it, the more he realized the two-minute lesson he'd inadvertently received in the spring was not sufficient.

After six months on the waiting list for mobility training, Kevin was finally assigned an instructor. He was delighted when Annie called to set up their first appointment. He was also filled with anxiety.

Coordination had never been Kevin's strong suit, even before he became blind. He was not a natural born athlete. As he waited for Annie's arrival, painful flashbacks to his less than illustrious Little League baseball career played in his mind. At the insistence of his father, who had been both assistant coach and umpire on different occasions, Kevin joined Little League and endured three years of profound humiliation in center field. Before he'd made a single play, his ill-fitting uniform already told the world just how unsuited he was for the sport. His gray jersey, in the largest available size, clung to his overweight body like the casing on a pork sausage. The fire engine red cap was so tight that it balanced precariously atop his head.

As he waited for his first appointment with Annie, Kevin was haunted by memories of an ungainly eleven-year-old being verbally pummeled after his dismal performance contributed to yet another crushing loss for his team. In a strange nod to the future, the local beer distributor, Fazio's Beverages, had sponsored his team.

Faith came to the rescue again. She helped Kevin shift his focus from one of fear to one of confidence. He was soon able to look at learning to use the cane from a different point of view—not as something that was forced upon him like baseball, rather as something he was choosing to do in order to gain mobility in the world at large. This fresh outlook changed everything—no longer did he need to feel immobilized by his loss of sight because he was using his power to learn new ways of coping with it.

Even with this more positive perspective, Kevin still felt the need for two vodkas to fortify himself for his first lesson with Annie at 9 A.M. "It's a breakfast drink," he justified to himself, as he added a splash of grapefruit juice.

Annie arrived, and at Kevin's request, she offered him a description of her physical appearance.

"I'm African-American, about five feet three inches, medium frame, with curly hair and oval, copper-toned, wire-rimmed glasses. I usually carry a backpack filled to capacity. I left it downstairs because I just trotted up the three flights."

"Why in the world did you do that?" Kevin asked. Annie laughed in embarrassment.

"I'm afraid of elevators, and so I left my backpack with the doorman. I'm sure glad you don't live on a higher floor!" she said, chuckling.

Annie's admission of her own vulnerabilities helped to further calm Kevin's nerves. With the introductions behind them, Annie wasted no time getting down to business. After determining that Kevin was right-handed, Annie positioned his hand on the cane to demonstrate how it should be held.

"Your hand needs to grip the top of the cane and remain positioned in the center of your chest," Annie explained. She held her hand over Kevin's and gently tapped the cane, first to the left surface of the ground in front of Kevin's body, and then to the right.

"There is a rhythm to using a cane," she went on.

"Like ballroom dancing," Kevin suggested, echoing Henry's words.

"Yes, that's right. Something like that. Before you take a step with your left foot, the cane should be in front of your left foot and likewise before you step with your right."

Kevin thought that sounded easy enough. Annie also offered a newer technique, referred to as a "constant sweep" which involved a left to right motion on the surface of the ground, rather than tapping.

"I'd like you to master the tapping technique first, and then you can switch to the constant sweep method, if you prefer."

Annie's teaching style suited Kevin well—detailed descriptions delivered in a laid-back manner. The first three sessions were confined to the halls and stairwells of Kevin's apartment building. The fourth lesson took them to the streets, and Kevin was soon navigating the city sidewalks with ease. In fact, he was downright amazed at how comfortable he felt.

He was in charge again.

Annie explained that the cane is an effective tool that provides a wealth of information.

"It's similar to having a portable advance team at your service. The cane surveys the walking surface for direction, constantly alerting its user of impending danger—fire hydrants, scaffolding, construction sites, sidewalk obstructions, cracks, and holes, to name a few."

Kevin took to heart his lessons about the importance of practice. Each day he pushed himself to venture outdoors and go a little further than the day before. For the first time in his life, Kevin felt proficient at a physical activity.

If only his father could see him now!

SELECTED JOURNAL ENTRY:

October 4, 2014—today my view is much brighter. My eyes also seem more open; perhaps more light is getting in.

CHAPTER 11

A New Angle

Summer 1998

Like most of us, Kevin had taken his vision for granted. It had been a given, like air and water.

Kevin's eyesight, however, was more than the ability to see. He was blessed with a "good eye." He'd viewed life through a wide-angle lens—both literally and figuratively. Since acquiring his first 35mm Canon camera at the age of fifteen, a significant amount of his leisure time had been spent viewing the world through its lens. His eyes continually scanned the world for that perfect shot. He'd never quite known what his quirky, yet discerning, eye was looking for until the moment had been right—when the picture in his head coincided with what he saw through the viewfinder.

One of his favorite photographers, Robert Mapplethorpe, referred to this elusive point in time as "the perfect moment." Kevin was often looking for an angle or perspective that was not readily evident to the naked eye. He would study the subject, usually a building, at various times throughout the day, under different lighting conditions, and from different vantage points, until it felt just right.

His photograph of The Watergate in Washington, D.C. was an example of his quest for the perfect shot. This now notorious structure is a complex of three oblong 1960s-era buildings.

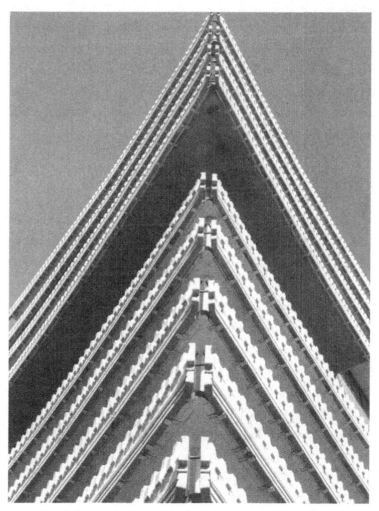

The Watergate. From Kevin's unique perspective.

For several days, Kevin had circled his favorite of the three buildings until the moment was just right—when ribbons of steel and molded concrete intersected on the side of the oval residential building. On the surface, the resulting graceful pagoda-like image he captured bared little resemblance to the iconic Washington landmark, yet it was exactly what Kevin had envisioned.

The perfect moment in time found Kevin lying on his back in between two rows of gas pumps at a station located two blocks away from The Watergate on Virginia Avenue. As he stretched out on the oil-slicked pavement, tilting his head back and forth waiting for the perfect perspective to enter the viewfinder, an impatient motorist honked furiously for him to move.

* * *

In addition to photography, Kevin's interest in the visual arts had led him to numerous museums. He'd been an enthusiastic and regular visitor to the exhibitions and retrospectives of the world's greatest photographers and artists.

Faith's perspective and encouragement gave him the courage to explore his love of visual arts once again. Given his penchant toward perfectionism, it was not surprising that he chose an ambitious goal for his first foray into this new way of looking at the world.

He decided to go to the Jackson Pollock retrospective at the Museum of Modern Art. Kevin had a strong affinity for Pollock's work. It angered him when the critics failed to see its merits, referring to his technique as random or happenstance. Kevin saw feeling and strong-willed volition in every splotch, drip, and splatter.

Kevin called MoMA and asked the switchboard operator to connect him with someone who had experience in providing visual descriptions of exhibits. Kevin attempted to explain his situation as briefly as possible.

"Good morning, I'd like to speak with someone with a high level of knowledge about Jackson Pollock's work. I have clear visual images of his paintings, but I've recently lost my sight. I was hoping there would be someone who could accompany me around the upcoming retrospective." Kevin was not surprised when the receptionist took the conversation in a different direction.

"You are more than welcome to come feel our Rockefeller sculpture collection," she offered. Kevin kept his cool but made no bones about his request.

"Let me try to better explain—I am looking for someone to provide a verbal description of the Jackson Pollock retrospective." She paused and attempted to process Kevin's unusual request.

"Hmm. Well, you could rent a cassette player with a pre-recorded commentary by a renowned art historian."

Kevin hung up the phone and picked up a glass.

Time for a vodka.

The next morning, bruised but not defeated, Kevin placed another call to MoMA and asked to be connected to the curatorial department. The operator informed him that their staff didn't speak directly to the public. However, she did agree to connect him to Guest Services instead.

"Good morning, Guest Services, how can I help you?" chirped a friendly female voice. Kevin explained his situation and repeated his request of the previous day. His second request met with the same offer of the sculpture collection. Kevin was disappointed but persisted.

"I understand that the curatorial staff does not generally speak to the public; perhaps you could intervene on my behalf and have someone call me back if there is any interest in helping me."

"By all means, sir, I will pass on your request."

Three weeks later, Kevin received an unexpected voice mail from a lady named Frances who introduced herself as an associate curator at MoMA. She sounded very friendly and said she would love to have the opportunity to fulfill his request. Kevin didn't waste a minute. He called her back and made an appointment to meet her the following week.

Frances greeted Kevin with cheerful enthusiasm and explained that they had a big challenge in front of them. Given that there were more than a hundred Pollock works spread out over seventeen galleries, it would be far too daunting to tackle each piece. Instead, Frances had chosen eighteen seminal works; each was a series of two or three pieces that was representative of a critical phase in Pollock's life.

Frances began their visit with a walking tour of the life-size, reconstructed Jackson Pollock studio in East Hampton. Pollock's actual studio had been in a barn, and the replicated one was appointed with wood planks that had been procured from a real barn. In the center on the floor was the signature twenty-foot-wide by fourteen-foot-high canvas that Pollock might have been working on. Kevin was able to walk through the studio and "feel" the presence of the artist in the space. He could imagine him walking around the huge canvas throwing paint here and there as he created his next masterpiece.

As Kevin took in the feel of the wood planks under his feet and the immense canvas that dominated the center of the studio, Frances told him the story of how Pollock had gotten his start with large canvases that would eventually become his trademark. He'd been living in a typical small New York City apartment when Peggy Guggenheim commissioned a large painting for the foyer of her New York City townhouse.

Too poor to afford a studio, Pollock painted in his living room. His living room was much too small to accommodate Peggy Guggenheim's commissioned painting. Pollock had a simple solution—he broke through his living room wall so that the work could extend into his tiny bedroom. Guggenheim loved his work, and Pollock soared into the top tier of the New York art world.

Frances spent the next three hours not only describing the physical attributes of each piece. She also provided the context as to how each was influenced by the psychological, romantic, and economic circumstances of the artist's life. Her detailed, well thought-out descriptions enabled Kevin to "see" each one of these complex paintings in his mind. However, her thoughtful commentary and astute observations had the greatest impact on Kevin.

"Pollock had an urgent drive to realize pictorial intensity at any price," Frances continued. "And he had a psychological need to cover every millimeter of the canvas with an intense physical energy that bore witness to his troubled soul."

The Pollock exhibit was a defining moment in Kevin's new life. It taught him that he could remain connected to the visual world, as long as he had the willingness to "see" it, as he had done with his photography, from a different angle.

However, with each situation, whether it was a theatre performance, an art exhibit, or something as mundane as clothes shopping, Kevin had to decide whether the benefit derived from receiving the verbal information outweighed the immense loss of not being able to see the object or event for himself.

SELECTED JOURNAL ENTRY:

November 4, 2014—today I am adding a new concoction to my recuperative regime. I am drinking honey and milk. Taken together, they form a powerful antioxidant that has been used by many cultures for centuries. As the saying goes—"it couldn't hurt."

CHAPTER 12

Les

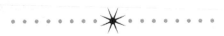

Fall 1998

One afternoon following another enjoyable and productive counseling session with Faith, Kevin left the Guild to begin his trip home. His journey had become routine. He got off the bus from the west side and walked to Lexington Avenue to catch the downtown bus. The corner of 68th Street and Lexington was always very crowded because of its proximity to Hunter College.

Kevin swept the surface of the sidewalk with his cane, attempting to find the bus stop. He first encountered hordes of people rushing by, then obstacles like a trash can and a newspaper-dispensing box. To confirm that he was indeed at the bus stop, he used his hands and followed the pole upward to the long rectangular sign.

The bus arrived, and Kevin boarded it. As he put his MetroCard in the slot, he asked the driver if he could please tell him when they got to 37th Street. Kevin located his customary seat behind the driver and was soon greeted by a friendly voice.

"How are you doing today? I want to say that I was pretty impressed with how you found the bus stop amongst all that mishegas."

Kevin normally didn't speak with strangers on the bus, but he was drawn to this man who radiated not only a warmth and compassion toward Kevin, but an interest, as well.

"Thank you. I'm still in the process of learning to use the cane."

"I had a hunch that you were pretty new at this, and you really did a great job," the man said enthusiastically.

The conversation continued as if they were old pals, and Kevin was really enjoying it. As the bus approached Kevin's destination, the man introduced himself.

"My name is Les, by the way. I've really enjoyed meeting you. If you give me your number, I'd like to call you tonight and continue our conversation." Kevin wasn't in the habit of handing out his phone number, nevertheless, it just felt right to do so this time.

True to his word, Les called that evening. Kevin was not a big phone person. Five hours later, he found himself still engaged in active conversation about personal histories to nutrition and spirituality. Of significant importance, Les was also gay, a fact Kevin had discerned even before he'd gotten off the bus.

Their bond was deep and immediate. Within a few weeks, Kevin and Les were a couple, Kevin's only significant relationship since college. A month later, Les moved into Kevin's apartment. Although Kevin enjoyed their physical relationship, of far more importance was that Les affirmed that Kevin was still a desirable man, despite his blindness.

Les was encouraging, constantly telling Kevin that his courage was an inspiration to him, as well as, to others. He was kind and loving, not only to Kevin, but also to random strangers they would meet on the streets during their outings. He would often carry food in his backpack on their walks and hand it out to the homeless. They enjoyed the city's varied and seemingly endless things to do, including museum hopping, going to restaurants or parks or simply taking in the energy of the bustling urban nightlife.

Both fans of Yiddish words, Les surprised Kevin one day with a Yiddish dictionary that he would read to Kevin on many evenings when they decided to stay home and take it easy. It was the kind of simple fun that helped deepen their relationship.

Les was an avid meditation and yoga enthusiast, and Kevin was inspired by his commitment. During those first months of their relationship, Kevin took his first baby steps toward developing his own practice. He would wake up before dawn and sit in silence for several hours. It was the only quiet time available before the busy New York streets came to life.

Kevin's initial foray into his meditation practice was not atypical. He noticed random thoughts entering his head. Kevin would observe them and then return to his breathing or mantra. When he complained that he "wasn't any good at meditation," Les was quick to encourage him.

"Just stick with it. You'll get."

There was one thing, however, that Les made very clear that he did not like about Kevin.

His drinking.

"Why do you need that drink?" Les would ask repeatedly.

Kevin always had the same answer.

"My life is very stressful."

"Everyone's life is stressful in one way or the other. That's not a justification for your daily consumption of large amounts of booze."

"I'm blind. Leave me alone."

Les wouldn't argue with him, but Kevin did not stop (or even cut back) on his drinking. Nevertheless, despite the friction over the drinking issue, for the first several months of their relationship, Kevin began to almost feel normal again.

However, the tension in their relationship was soon apparent. The more Kevin drank, the more Les retreated into his meditation and yoga interests. Kevin did his best to emulate his friend, to put meditating before drinking. He just couldn't do it. Kevin loved Les, but he loved vodka more.

One morning, without warning, explanation or fanfare, Les announced that he was leaving.

"I'm moving to a meditation and yoga community in Fairfield, Iowa."

Kevin was surprised and not surprised at the same time. He put his coffee mug on the kitchen counter, stood up and walked into the living room to turn on some music. Despite the announcement, Kevin was grateful for all the acceptance and love Les had showered upon him in their short time together. Most important, the commitment Les demonstrated to his yoga and meditation practice would one day catapult Kevin into his own journey of inner transformation.

When Les walked out of the apartment, it was a bittersweet moment. Kevin felt both sad and relieved.

Now, he could drink as much as he wanted again, without observation or comment.

SELECTED JOURNAL ENTRY:

December 14, 2014—someone on the street remarks that my facial expression looks quite different. I ask her to explain. She states that I look much lighter and more alive!

CHAPTER 13

Wardrobe Madness

Winter 1999

Kevin's clothes-consciousness throughout his adult life was rooted in the awful childhood experiences of being outfitted in The Husky Shop. Although grateful for the stored visual memories of his youth, he would have been happy to delete that particular image from his memory bank. As a blind person, developing a system for organizing his clothes was a lengthy and tedious process. Kevin was an orderly person who lived his life free of clutter and that made his task much easier. Pablo's advice—organization and placement—provided the foundation for Kevin's system, and, and with the help of several sighted friends, he started by grouping all similar items together.

In addition, he derived inspiration from several other friends. Dorothy, his mother's good friend who had been born blind, taught Kevin how to place safety pins and beads in labels to differentiate garments. Another friend, a clothing designer, provided adhesive Velcro tabs of every size, shape, and texture to place on labels.

Kevin lined up dress shirts by color and pattern (white, pink, striped, checked). He arranged his dress trousers by material type (wool, khaki, linen). He grouped his casual clothing in a similar manner— jeans, sweaters, black t-shirts, white t-shirts, and polo shirts.

Within each subcategory, Kevin differentiated colors by placement of safety pins and Velcro tabs—one safety pin for orange clothing, two safety pins for pink, one safety pin with a bead for burgundy, one safety pin with two beads for green, textured Velcro for black and soft Velcro for navy blue.

The system required vigilance. He could not put things away haphazardly. He had to return everything to its exact place after wearing or laundering.

Regular grooming practices like shaving, bathing and brushing teeth were less difficult, and within a few months, Kevin had mastered them all. The biggest challenge was that every single task took at least three times longer to complete—not easy for someone who had always been impatient and fast-paced.

While learning to dress and groom himself required practice and patience, learning to navigate the streets of New York City required a different set of adaptations.

First, Kevin needed to maximize his hearing by any means necessary. Even though Kevin's hearing did not improve when he lost his sight, he relied on it far more. Discovering that head coverings tended to mute sound, Kevin went bareheaded, whatever the weather. He donated all of his hats, caps and hoodies to charity.

One of the more difficult tasks for Kevin to master was dialing a phone. He replaced his sleek Bang & Olufsen with an old-fashioned touch-tone with buttons. It took countless hours of practice over the course of months to develop the proper rhythm. Using the five as a reference point (old touch-tone phones had a raised mark on the five key), he counted up, down, and over to dial numbers. He had some interesting conversations with strangers he had misdialed!

Another task that was not easy for Kevin to master was learning to type again. Even using a pen and paper was difficult. Typing was harder. Hunt and peck—two-finger typing and searching for the keys by sight—doesn't work well for a blind man.

The Jewish Guild for the Blind provided Kevin with a private typing tutor, Audrey, who was blind from birth. She gave Kevin an old typewriter that she'd schlepped on Metro North from her home in Westchester. They quickly became friends, and Kevin even received a wet kiss from her German Shepard guide dog.

From their first visit, despite her pleasant manner, Audrey was anxious to get down to business.

"Okay, I am going to place your fingers on the all-important home row," she explained.

With her hands on top of Kevin's, their fingers moved together across the keyboard in perfect synchronicity. Audrey's patience put Kevin at ease. In no time, he was practicing three hours a day and looking forward to their next session. Within five months, he was able to type twenty-five words per minute with a high degree of accuracy.

Kevin's practice sessions were made easier due to the generosity of a friend who bought him his first computer. Another friend, a Radford fraternity brother, organized a fund-raising drive to buy the computer text-to-speech software that enabled the computer to read out loud.

However, like many people who experience adult-onset blindness, Kevin was not able to master Braille, even after many months of instruction. While he learned to distinguish fabrics by the mere touch of his finger, because his appearance remained important to him, he wasn't that interested in reading Braille or any activity strictly associated with being blind. Despite the undeniable fact that Kevin was indeed blind, he persisted in fighting against this reality with every ounce of his will.

* * *

A few months after Kevin had managed to relearn these daily activities, he received a call from a rehabilitation counselor who was mandated by New York State to visit him in his home once a week for the next ten weeks to make sure he was safe. Kevin was not pleased by the timing.

"Are you kidding me?" he shouted into the phone. "I needed your help more than a year ago, not now!" This must have been a typical response because the rehabilitation counselor remained calm.

"Sir, you sound very angry." The counselor paused, clearly waiting for a response from Kevin. When he didn't get one—Kevin was quietly pouring a drink—he continued.

"Are you receiving mental health services?" The vodka served its purpose and Kevin remained unfazed.

"I'm not angry or mentally impaired—just remarkably resourceful, and I no longer need your help."

"That's all well and good, sir, but I'm required by New York state law to make sure you're safe in your home." By now Kevin had learned that it was always futile, and often detrimental, to fight the system so they arranged their first visit for the following week.

Kevin served the counselor hot tea and slices of cheddar cheese. This satisfied the requirement of demonstrating that he could safely boil water and use a sharp knife. He passed the home exam, and the counselor told him he didn't need to take the "Cutting Carrots 101" class at the Guild. "What a relief, no carrot chopping," thought Kevin sarcastically, as he closed the door on the counselor.

Learning to perform daily activities without sight was much easier for Kevin than confronting the lingering emotions surrounding his blindness. Despite countless cups of spilled coffee, navigating his new external world was far easier on every level than stepping a single foot into his internal one.

However, Kevin slowly began to cultivate the ability to confront this new world. His initial reaction was to lash out. Over time, that attitude softened. He was now on a parallel journey to freedom that didn't depend on his intellect, will, or reason.

Or even on his sight.

SELECTED JOURNAL ENTRY:

January 29, 2015—my field of vision is much brighter. Additionally, from time to time, I experience flashes of blue and green.

CHAPTER 14

Lost and Found

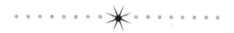

Spring 1999

Kevin had been blind for two years. It was long enough to go without a guide dog, however, there was one large obstacle standing in his way—his beloved Weimaraner, Pepper.

It was a cold night in February 1990 when Kevin had picked her up from Washington National airport. He'd found her through an advertisement in the *Washington Post*, placed by a breeder in Laredo, Texas. Pepper was ten months old when Kevin first met her that winter night. She was a beautiful dog with a velvety, medium-gray coat and gray-blue eyes. And she was already a giant.

Their first night together didn't go well. Pepper circled the living room for hours until she passed out from exhaustion. Kevin, exhausted himself, grabbed a blanket and spent that first night on his living room floor right beside her. By morning, Kevin and Pepper had bonded.

D.C. was a culture shock for Pepper—from the wide, open spaces of a Texas ranch to the smaller space of Kevin's first-floor, two-bedroom apartment in Logan Circle. Even the city's wide boulevards could not replace the space and freedom Pepper had enjoyed on the ranch.

During the first two weeks, Pepper destroyed Kevin's LL Bean's moccasins, six plastic CD cases, two large fireplace logs, two Swatch watches, speaker wires, phone lines, and untold numbers of books and magazines. Kevin's roommate's possessions weren't safe either. She ate his Rolling Stone magazine in the short time he left it on the sofa while making coffee.

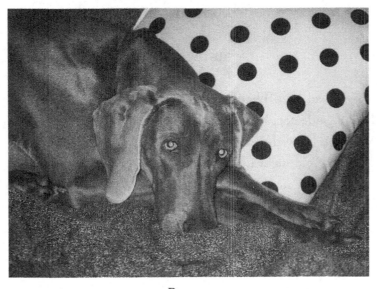

Pepper

Pepper seemed to know what she was after. Even after weeks of training, Kevin returned home from work and found his book by Barbara Woodhouse, *No Bad Dogs*, destroyed! Kevin couldn't help himself—he laughed out loud so long that his roommate thought something bad had happened. Nothing was off limits for Pepper—the chewing machine!

Then one day, without reason or explanation, Pepper stopped chewing. Even though her chewing had stopped, Kevin's roommate still insisted that they lock her in their spacious kitchen before leaving for their respective jobs in the morning. This plan seemed to be working well until one evening when Kevin returned home and found his kitchen door off its hinges lying on the floor. A short investigation led Kevin to his living room—Pepper was lounging on the living room sofa smiling. Fortunately, Pepper soon learned to open doors with her mouth, rather than knocking them down, so the rest of Kevin's doors and hinges were spared.

Most important, Pepper was fiercely loyal and devoted to Kevin. She was very much a one-person dog, as Weimaraners are known to be. It had not been an easy decision to give her up. Two large dogs in a tiny studio apartment, however, was not viable. Kevin had even managed to teach himself how to walk Pepper with his left hand while holding his cane in his right. Despite not being a guide dog, Pepper had been so in tune with him that she somehow sensed that he could no longer see, and she intuitively slowed her normal fast pace down a notch or two. Fortunately for Kevin, she also gave up her practice of stalking birds and squirrels.

At one point, Kevin felt he could almost get by with Pepper in place of a seeing-eye dog. Pepper was a lot of things, but she was not a trained guide dog. In the end, almost was almost. Reluctantly, Kevin gave her to his mobility instructor, Annie, and her roommate, Dorothy. He tried to set aside his sadness and loss and be grateful for all the joy Pepper had given him.

All seemed well for a week. Then Annie called.

"Kevin, you have to come take Pepper back immediately."

"Why, what's wrong?"

"She's not getting along at all with Dorothy's cat."

Kevin knew that if he took Pepper back he would never be able to give her up a second time. At Kevin's suggestion, Annie drove Pepper to the Yankee Woods Weimaraner Rescue League in Plymouth, Massachusetts.

She was soon adopted by a loving couple who called Kevin over the next year on a routine basis to let him know how Pepper was doing. She lived five more years to the age of fifteen, a long life for such a large dog.

Now without a dog, Kevin waited for the phone call that would change his life.

SELECTED JOURNAL ENTRY:

February 25, 2015—my world, long shuttered, is creeping into focus. I am allowing myself for the first time to visualize myself joyfully photographing all of the skyscrapers that have been built in the last eighteen years.

CHAPTER 15

Rugged Ruger

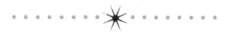

Summer 1999

Support groups, counselors, and canes were great, but what Kevin needed most of all was a seeing-eye dog. He'd tried to get by without one, but after finally making the decision to find Pepper a new home, Kevin applied for his first guide dog at The Seeing Eye and patiently waited his turn.

The call finally came.

The Seeing Eye organization started in Europe in the 1920s when American socialite Dorothy Harrison Eustis moved to Switzerland to set up a breeding and training facility for German Shepherds to assist German soldiers who had lost their sight during the First World War. She believed that guide dogs could have a wider potential for helping all visually impaired people.

She wrote an article for *The Saturday Evening Post* about her viewpoint on this important subject, published on November 5, 1927. Soon thereafter, Eustis began receiving letters from people who wanted her to train a dog for them. The first man she helped was Morris Frank, who lived in Nashville, and would later partner with her in founding The Seeing Eye in 1929.

The Seeing Eye was the first guide dog school outside of Europe, and it is now the oldest existing school in the world. It matches more than 250 visually impaired people each year with guide dogs. There are currently more than 1,700 Seeing Eye dog users in the United States and Canada. The Seeing Eye moved in 1931 from its original home in Nashville to Whippany, NJ and then again in 1965 to a modern, facility in Morris Township, NJ.

When the call that Kevin had been waiting for finally came, he was anxious. Judy, the head of admissions introduced herself. She had barely finished her preliminary remarks when Kevin interrupted her.

"When can I get my dog?"

"First, we have to schedule a face-to-face interview with a trainer. Your instructor will be Shannon."

"I'm ready! When can I meet her? Will she bring a dog?" Kevin asked, his impatience clearly evident.

"No, you'll meet a dog here in Morristown. First, there will be an interview in your home. Then Shannon will take you on a Juno Walk, and she'll explain more about that when you meet. This is to help measure your strength, gait and walking speed, and acquaint you with the harness."

"When can I start?" Kevin was getting more and more excited. He had seen first-hand the difference seeing-eye dogs had made in the lives of his friends in the support group. Ken and Bill often brought their dogs, Garrick and Smitty, to group meetings.

Shannon arranged to come to New York City the following week. After a brief question and answer session, Shannon was ready to take Kevin out onto the sidewalks. Shannon acted the role of the guide dog with the harness strapped around her waist. While it was all a bit comical and embarrassing, Shannon urged Kevin to relax.

"Just have some fun. I know it's a little weird, but this is an essential diagnostic tool in matching an applicant with the right dog."

Shannon and Kevin were soon out on Park Avenue. While Shannon was playing the part of guide dog, Kevin was the one barking orders.

"Faster, slower," Kevin said. He could not keep from laughing at the situation and himself. He was indeed having fun.

The exercise continued for forty-five minutes until Shannon was confident that she'd collected the necessary data. In addition to strength, gait and walking speed, Shannon also took careful notes about Kevin's neighborhood, lifestyle, and personality. Once she had all her data points, Shannon and Kevin headed back to his apartment.

"Kevin, we're about halfway there," she explained. "Although much of the process of matching students with potential dogs takes place during the application process, the final decision is not made until the point students are formally introduced to their new partners. I'm going to take all this information back to the school, and someone will call you when it's time for the next step."

"How long will that take?" Kevin asked nervously.

"Several months," Shannon explained.

"Several months!" Kevin shouted. "I've already been waiting several months."

"I understand the process is long and frustrating, Kevin, but it's important to make the right match so the dogs do not have to be returned."

* * *

A few months later, Kevin finally received a call from The Seeing Eye. He wasted no time in heading to Morristown to begin the month-long training process. During the first two days of class, the staff observed how the students interacted with a variety of potential candidates before they finalized their decision.

A few days later, Kevin sat in an overstuffed wing chair in the tastefully appointed lounge, named for Eustis, who had endowed the school with five million dollars in her will.

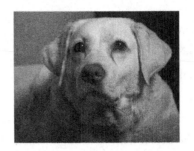

He waited anxiously to meet the guide dog Shannon had selected for him. Kevin was sweating; he'd gone on the wagon before heading out to the school and was feeling the effects of sudden alcohol withdrawal.

His anxiety, as well as his sweating, abated when he sensed an enormous, fluffy presence that Shannon introduced as Ruger.

"Kevin, I have someone I would like you to meet." Kevin got down on the floor and was greeted with a big wet lick on the face.

"This is Ruger. He has a very handsome face. He has amber colored eyes, accentuated by beautiful dark-brown lashes—he actually looks like he is wearing eyeliner!" Shannon joked. "He's a big, yellow Lab with a strong jaw and a huge, square head, weighing in at 68 pounds!"

The next step was to take the training class. Each class included twenty-five students who were broken up into smaller groups of four, headed by its own instructor. During the first week, the focus was on orienting the students to the floor plan of the dormitory and becoming acquainted with the training staff and other classmates. It was also a time for the students to begin bonding with their guide dogs. From the time students and dogs were introduced, they are required to be together around the clock.

Kevin soon found himself out on the local streets of Morristown, navigating a variety of pre-selected routes. The first two days, Kevin walked with his instructor following close behind. On the third day, he was required to complete the course solo.

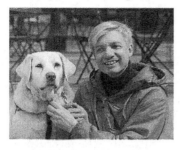

While the students were learning to navigate downtown Morristown, the senior instructor was circling in a van. His goal was not only to observe the behavior of the students and their dogs, but also to provide "traffic checks." The term refers to cars turning in front of a student and dog team as they are crossing an intersection, or cars turning out of a driveway or exiting a parking lot; in other words, practice in a controlled setting presenting real life, potentially dangerous situations.

One day, Ruger and Kevin were waiting at a corner when the senior instructor turned his van right in front of them.

Ruger did his job and stopped short.

Kevin didn't.

Ruger ignored Kevin's command to go forward. Kevin became impatient, dropped his harness, and proceeded into the street without him.

"Hey, Mr. New York, you need to trust your dog," shouted the instructor. "Stop being a maniac New Yorker and let your dog lead you."

That day Kevin learned two of the cardinal rules when working with a guide dog. One, never drop the harness, particularly not at an intersection, and two, always trust your dog. Kevin set his own cockiness aside and did everything the instructor and Ruger told him. He passed all three of his next solo route tests with top marks.

* * *

Kevin returned home with Ruger the following week. He chose an ambitious route for their first walk. They caught the bus up Madison

Avenue and then transferred to the crosstown bus at 66th Street. They got off at Central Park West and crossed to the southwest corner of the intersection.

Ruger abruptly stopped. Kevin gave Ruger a forward command, but Ruger resisted. Kevin gave him a "hup up" command meaning to speed it up. Ruger stood firm. Once again, Kevin gave the "hup up" command. Ruger proceeded forward two steps, and Kevin went head first into a ladder that was leaning out from some scaffolding, cutting his forehead right above his left eye. From that day on, whenever Ruger encountered scaffolding (a frequent occurrence in New York City) he just sat down and refused to walk through it. Kevin got frustrated by this but finally realized he was the problem, not Ruger.

The main challenge had nothing to do with whether Kevin believed Ruger could do his job or not. The difficulty that Kevin had letting Ruger in on an emotional level—allowing total trust to develop between them—was partly due to the deep connection he still felt with Pepper.

Although he'd found Pepper a good home and knew on an intellectual level that he could no longer provide her with the exercise she craved, he still resented the fact that he'd had to give her up. Pepper was the first dog that Kevin had truly loved, and she had been his loyal and constant companion for eight years. Although Kevin had desperately wanted, and was excited about having, a seeing-eye dog, he couldn't help feeling some resentment toward Ruger.

And it wasn't just that Ruger wasn't Pepper. He realized he was resenting Ruger for what he represented—Kevin's blindness. Even though Kevin had accepted his blindness by now, he still found physical manifestations of this difficult to accept. A guide dog was like a white cane to Kevin. He felt that both, while useful and even necessary, screamed out "blind man on board."

On occasion, Kevin also had to deal with people's overblown expectations of what a guide dog can do. A couple of months after returning home with Ruger, Kevin was at a friend's house in East Hampton, Long Island at a dinner party. During the meal, a woman seated to his left tapped him on the shoulder.

"Does he answer the phone for you?" she asked in a serious tone.

"Not only does he answer the phone, in a voice reminiscent of Astro from The Jetsons, he also handles all my scheduling and makes a superb bacon and cheese omelet."

Kevin didn't actually say that but wanted to do so.

"No," Kevin replied politely instead. "He just guides me around New York City."

This kind of ignorance had the effect of encouraging Kevin to defend his dog, and at last, he forged a strong connection with Ruger. Like a dance team, they developed their own rhythm in tune with the city.

An unexpected deepening in their relationship finally came the day Ruger expressed frustration with tourists. Kevin and Ruger were walking through the heart of Times Square. As they proceeded westward, crowds of sluggish pedestrians blocked their way. Ruger first tried to go around to the left, then to the right. Unable to clear a path through the sea of humanity, he began to stomp his paws in place.

Kevin suddenly loved him unconditionally. Ruger had become an impatient New Yorker just like him!

SELECTED JOURNAL ENTRY:

March 13, 2015—I'm still using my cane, but it is so freeing to almost see my way as I briskly walk up Park Avenue, and then head east on 34th Street.

CHAPTER 16

Pencil Man

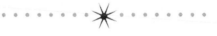

Spring 2000

The spring was slow in coming. After being stuck inside for much of the winter, Kevin was anxious to resume his three-mile daily outings with Ruger. Kevin didn't mind the cold, but the icy New York City sidewalks were treacherous for everyone, especially a blind man. Ruger was an exceptional guide dog, still there was a limit to his ability to navigate around the large snow mounds that often blocked the intersections.

When those first welcome spring days arrived, Kevin wasted no time getting back out onto the streets with Ruger. Kevin liked to walk a large quadrant route that started at his apartment building, went westward to Fifth Avenue, up to 57th Street, East to Lexington, and then back downtown again. He encountered occasional difficulties. Navigating the city blocks, and even the city traffic, were the least of them.

New Yorkers, who often meant well, were sometimes insensitive. Kevin was blind, but he was not otherwise disabled, and obviously his intelligence had not been affected by his loss of sight. If anything, Kevin was now much more in tune with his environment. When pedestrians

78

assumed he was lost, Kevin would quite often get infuriated. On the other hand, people's beliefs that guide dogs were imbued with human-like abilities, was equally upsetting to him.

One day, Kevin's frustration reached new heights when he and Ruger were waiting on the corner of Madison Avenue and 41ˢᵗ Street for the light to change. A guide dog, like all dogs, has a very limited ability to distinguish colors. Hence, the perception that a guide dog can alert his master when traffic lights change color is a false one. Rather, a blind person becomes aware of the shifting sounds of traffic patterns, in order to determine when parallel traffic begins to flow. It is the handler who gives the guide dog a verbal forward command when it is safe to proceed. Although guide dogs do learn frequently traveled routes, as well as to pause in front of familiar locations, the reality is they don't move forward without the specific command to do so.

A few seconds after the northbound light turned red and the traffic stopped, Kevin was about to give Ruger the forward signal when a pedestrian pushed roughly past him.

"Hey mister, your dog isn't doing his job properly. The light is green." The man was gone before Kevin could answer. He seethed with anger instead.

A few blocks farther north, still cursing under his breath, Kevin lost count of which street he was on. As he waited on the next corner, he asked the person standing to his left, "Excuse me, sir, are we on the corner of Madison and Forty-Fourth or Forty-Fifth?"

"Ask your guide dog," the man answered brusquely. "Can't he tell you?"

The rage Kevin felt for the next few blocks dissipated when he found himself in front of Saks Fifth Avenue. It brought back fond memories of his first job after college. Kevin had worked just a few blocks away for Mutual of America, a well-known insurance company. Even though he could only afford to buy a shirt or tie at Saks now and then, he nevertheless liked to frequent the store on his lunch breaks. As Kevin paused to reflect on this part of his life, he heard the familiar voice of an old man calling out to people going in and out of the store.

"Pencils for sale! Pencils for sale!" The man had become a fixture outside of Saks many years earlier and sold pencils for five cents day in, day out, rain or shine. He was blind.

Kevin remembered how he'd always bought a pencil from him each time he visited Saks on his lunch hour, whether he needed one or not. Kevin had always felt sorry for the man. That day Kevin bought another pencil that he didn't need, but he did not feel sorry for him. As he dropped his nickel in the man's cup, he said, "Thank you for the pencil. Have a good day, sir."

Viewed through his own blindness, and with his recent unfortunate encounters in the street fresh in his mind, Kevin saw the man in a new way. He was out there in the real world. Getting on with his life. Living it the best way he could. Ignoring ignorant people. And he had the ingenuity to make a living despite his disability. That deserved Kevin's admiration and praise, not pity. That day, Kevin took another step forward in his inner transformation. His view of life and people was changing.

There was still one important thing Kevin still needed to do. And that one challenge would prove to be his most difficult. As is often the case when we are faced with life's most difficult obstacles, Kevin would have to overcome it alone.

April 28, 2015—today is characterized by intense activity in my head and face. First of all, I feel an unrelenting pain on the left side of my forehead. As I lay in bed, I experience continual, yet gentle, throbbing throughout my face, but it is most pronounced directly under my eyes.

CHAPTER 17

Bent Knees

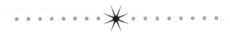

Winter 2001

Life can be divided into the before and after of major milestones—leaving home for college, graduation, marriage, divorce, children.

One of Kevin's critical dividing lines was January 21, 2001.

The night before, Kevin had arranged to meet friends in Chelsea. He was on 14th Street and Ninth Avenue. With fifteen minutes to pass, he reclined against a storefront with Ruger stretched out comfortably on the sidewalk in front of him. His momentary calm was soon interrupted by a woman's voice.

"You must be lost. You must be looking for that building on Twenty-Third Street where all the blind people live." Kevin had been drinking in his apartment during the course of the day. This caused him to be more snarky than usual in his response.

"Excuse me, I would have to be not just blind but totally clueless to be standing on Fourteenth Street and Ninth Avenue and be looking for a building that is located on Twenty-Third Street between Sixth and Seventh Avenues!" The woman stormed off without saying another word.

When Kevin woke the next day, the woman and his reaction to her were the first things that crossed his mind. She was trying to be helpful. He saw her as being rude, interfering, and patronizing. And that perception was in no small part driven by the alcohol he had consumed.

The scenario played over and over in his mind throughout the morning. He'd been drunk and subsequently rude to people before, of course, but this time, it haunted him.

Kevin knew that people who struggled with addiction, could be presented with a chance to get sober. Some referred to these as "moments of grace." Others called them "windows of opportunity." Some people grabbed them. Some didn't recognize the moments, and they passed by.

That moment for Kevin happened following the delivery of his booze later that afternoon. Kevin no longer walked to the liquor store. He didn't attempt to struggle uphill with booze in one hand and his cane in the other. And he didn't think it was proper to have Ruger guide him to his vodka supply. So he had started having his vodka delivered. His new supplier advertised warehouse prices and that suited Kevin just fine. No longer able to afford his favorite brand—Stoli—his standing order was for two plastic bottles of rot-gut vodka—$14.06 a half-gallon, two to three times a week. Not the smoothest vodka in the world, but it did the trick.

As soon as he heard the thud of the bottles being deposited in front of his door, he took them in and hid them in his coat closet, as always—one in a duffle bag on the floor, the other in a backpack hanging from a hook.

He couldn't remember when the secrecy had started. Maybe when he'd been trying to hide the volume of vodka he drank from Les. As Kevin was wrestling to get a bottle into his duffel bag, he was suddenly seized with emotion.

"What in the hell is wrong with this picture?" he said aloud. "Who am I hiding this from? I live alone, and I'm blind to boot." Kevin fell to his knees and began to cry violently.

He knew he had to be ashamed of his drinking on some level, otherwise why would he be hiding bottles? He knew deep down that his "friend" was no longer his friend. In that moment, Kevin felt his shame transform into motivation. He wanted to stop drinking. But he wasn't sure how to do it.

Kevin remembered that his business associate Dave had become sober several years earlier. He could talk to him. He called and left a message on Dave's voice mail before he changed his mind. Dave returned the call quickly.

"Hey Kevin, Dave here. I'm in New Orleans on business, and I'll be back next Sunday. What's up?"

"I really need some help," Kevin confessed without hesitation. "I'm an alcoholic."

"I can suggest some good meetings, if you're ready," Dave offered.

"Great, but I don't feel comfortable going by myself," Kevin admitted.

"I'll be back in time for the Sunday meeting that I chair; can you meet me then?" Dave asked.

"Fine, when and where?" Kevin asked.

"Do you have a way of taking down the information? I'll give you the address right now."

Kevin didn't hesitate; he reached for his cassette recorder.

SELECTED JOURNAL ENTRY:

May 27, 2015—at night, I am experiencing intense pain in the left side of my face. It is evident that long dormant nerves are firing up. The sensation is similar to what I remember feeling many years ago with an abscessed wisdom tooth.

CHAPTER 18

The Bowery

Spring 2001

Even though Dave was out of town, he made himself available to speak with Kevin on the phone, day or night that week. While Kevin had Dave's ear, he still had to go through the painful detox process alone—he didn't have the insurance or the financial resources to cover the cost of checking himself into a rehab center.

As Kevin squirmed on the floor in full withdrawal, he comforted himself with the belief that he could quit. He'd been through this once before two years earlier when he'd weaned himself off Valium. Addicted to the drug for just five months, he nevertheless had been taking 50 milligrams a day when he realized that he had to quit. Determined to eliminate at least one of his addictions, he had become Valium-free in eight days. This had been no small accomplishment, and Kevin knew he could do it again. He clenched his fists and gritted his teeth in preparation for the battle that lay ahead.

After twenty years of daily drinking it was a shock to Kevin's system to suddenly be cut off from the fuel it craved. During the first few days his body screamed out for its familiar fix. His hands trembled uncontrollably, and his stomach growled and constricted in painful spasms. He experienced chills followed by cold sweats. He left his apartment only to take Ruger to the sidewalk to relieve himself.

Kevin quickly lost twenty pounds, most of it within the first week, due in large part to his body shedding the bloating effect of alcohol. The fact that he was too nauseous to eat, accelerated his weight loss. Because of his determination, the intellectual component of getting sober was considerably easier than losing the physical compulsion to drink. Unable to afford even medicine, Kevin endured the initial withdrawal period without it.

Kevin couldn't wait for the Sunday meeting. He arrived at the location on Little West 12th Street twenty minutes early. He parked himself in front of the entrance, despite the cold. He was shaking and sweating even though it was January. He was contemplating returning to his apartment when he heard a cheerful voice call out.

"Hi, I'm Bob. Are you looking for the meeting?"

"Yes, I am. I'm Kevin, and this is my guide dog, Ruger."

"Great, come on in," Bob said with a kind and reassuring voice. Ruger, always a good judge of character, seemed to take an instant liking to Bob.

Bob introduced Kevin to the other early arrivals in the room. Dave arrived a few minutes later. Everyone was warm and gracious. They all spoke the same word—welcome.

Once the meeting got started, the speaker was introduced and greeted by applause. She told her story of being raised by Norwegian immigrant parents in a rural farming community in upstate New York. She described the trauma of losing her mother at a young age and how that had shaped her.

Though Kevin couldn't relate to any of the specifics of her life, he nonetheless felt a deep association with her pain. The details of their respective upbringings could not have been more different, and yet he had experienced the same underlying feelings she powerfully described—never fitting in, constantly feeling different and out of place and not knowing why. She explained that at first she drank to be more social and fit in; later she used drinking to numb her feelings of loss or pain. His drinking history was identical.

Kevin knew that this group was just what he needed. He'd long believed that his disposition toward alcoholism was preordained. There was a family history with the disease. Even though Kevin did not drink in high school, he'd had some sips from his grandfather's beer can while sitting on his lap as a child. He liked the taste of it, as well as, the warm fuzzy feeling it gave him. Even at that early age, Kevin craved more.

Kevin's next taste of alcohol had occurred at age ten, when he volunteered to play bartender for a small gathering of his mom's friends. After his mother instructed him on how to measure out scotch and whiskey sour mix, he eschewed the shot glass in favor of the heavy-handed pour. When no one was looking, he stole a few furtive slurps of his concoctions. He believed he was already a master bartender.

Kevin's drink of choice was always "more." Once he started the process by taking that first real drink in college, it was always about the next, and the next, and the next. As he began his journey of sobriety at age thirty-nine, learning that there were countless others who shared his same feelings was both validating and comforting.

Kevin had always experienced low self-esteem coupled with grandiosity and a huge sense of entitlement. Kevin heard person after person share the same dichotomous feelings. One speaker summed it up best.

"I felt like the biggest piece of shit that the entire universe revolved around."

Kevin left that afternoon a changed man and could not wait to attend the next meeting. The group gave him renewed hope. Each story of triumph over adversity bolstered his confidence that he too would succeed in becoming and remaining sober. Each member's story had its unique details, experiences, and geographic setting; at the same time, all had the common elements of pain, loss, despair, and ultimately, hope and triumph.

Kevin learned that alcoholism cut across all groups regardless of age, sex, ethnic origin, or socio-economic status. Whether people lived on Park Avenue or a park bench, their pain was the same. Kevin gained strength and hope from their diverse stories.

Up until then, Kevin had never thought of himself as an alcoholic. He knew he drank too much, and at times had lost his dignity as a result. Still, he felt his behavior fell into the "normal drinking range." To him, an alcoholic was someone who had lost everything and was living on Skid Row in Los Angeles or the Bowery in New York City. One story forever changed Kevin's view of what it meant to be an alcoholic.

One night, a serene man with thirty years of sobriety spoke of having once been a naval officer. He'd not only thrown away a promising military career, he'd also found himself living on the Bowery.

He recounted living on the street panhandling to get his next fix of wine or malt liquor. With great emotion, he explained how his journey of recovery had begun when a sober friend found him on the street and brought him to his first meeting. Kevin was stunned into silence, but another group member spoke up.

"I may have had a problem with alcohol, but at least I was never living on the Bowery." The ex-naval officer was polite but direct.

"My dear, the Bowery is not a place, it is a state of mind. Whenever and wherever an alcoholic experiences the demoralizing shame of not remembering what happened the night before, they are experiencing their own personal bowery." Kevin understood.

Kevin found hope and inspiration from others who had enjoyed long-term sobriety. His friends Bob, Michael, Barbara, Jane, and Sterling were his sober role models. When he asked them how they had done it, their advice was always the same and quite simple.

"Don't drink, go to meetings, and your life will begin to get better."

Alcohol had had a chokehold over him for the last twenty years. Kevin knew that it was going to be his determination coupled with the support of others that would lead him out of his drinking darkness.

Kevin did what they suggested, and within a few weeks things did start to improve. An unforeseen—yet critically important—gift of sobriety was Kevin's development of a relationship with a higher power. With a slow and begrudging realization, Kevin forged a relationship with a God of his own understanding.

There was a vast difference between that God and the one he'd known as a child. His Catholic school education had introduced Kevin to a vengeful, harsh, and unforgiving God. By contrast, the entity that Kevin now experienced was a loving, inclusive, and forgiving one. Kevin's higher power guided him, gave him strength, and kept him sober a day at a time.

Each morning, before he poured his first cup of coffee, Kevin got down on his knees and asked for the help of his higher power. His refrain was always the same.

"I can't. You can. Please help me to stay sober today."

During that daily ritual, despite his blindness, Kevin began by giving thanks for all the blessings of his life. And then he prayed for others. Kevin found that this switch from his self-concern to a focus on others, despite his own dire circumstances, was the single most defining perspective that changed his life.

Blind, broke, jobless, and frustrated, Kevin found it difficult to get through the next few months. But he had one big thing going for him.

He was sober.

Getting sober was both the best and the hardest thing that Kevin ever did. It was also the single one accomplishment of which he was, and remains, the proudest. It would also bring a gift, equal to, if not greater than, his sobriety.

It was a new beginning.

SELECTED JOURNAL ENTRY:

June 20, 2015—the throbbing in my forehead and under my eyes continues. I have to believe that it is a noteworthy occurrence, even though, recently, there is only a negligible improvement in my eyesight.

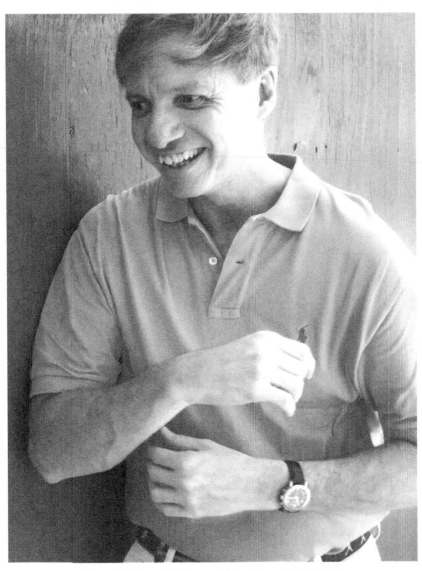

Kevin Coughlin, smiling again. NYC.

PART TWO

AMAZING GRACE

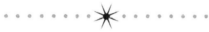

2001-2016

*"It is only with the heart that one can see wisely;
what is truly important in life is invisible to the eye."*
—Antoine de Saint-Exupery
The Little Prince

CHAPTER 19

Angels Among Us

Fall 2001

With sobriety, Kevin was able to face things that he'd hidden from himself during the years when he'd been drinking.

One of the first things he needed to do was get a job.

Dependent on his monthly social security disability check, as well as his parents' generosity, Kevin was ready to assume financial responsibility for himself once again.

Unemployment rates among the disabled were high, with the highest rate of all among the blind. Kevin knew that if he was ever going to work again, he not only needed to learn to type, he also had to learn to use the computer with proficiency.

Once again, the Jewish Guild for the Blind was there to help. Kevin set off for his first appointment with a man called Angel who would prove to be true to his name. The day did not get off to a good start, however.

On the bus headed uptown, Kevin located his customary seat behind the driver. As he was getting Ruger situated, it became clear that he was the topic of conversation between two elderly women across from him.

"Ida, you never know, you never know. Look at this young man." Ida responded in a loud gruff, New York City accent.

"It's true, you never know. I went to the eye doctor the other day. He checked the pressure. It was good, but you never know." Ida's friend chimed back in.

"It's such a shame. He is so young and good looking, but at least he has that smart dog. Those dogs are so amazing!"

Kevin felt his body tense up as he overheard their conversation. He wanted to speak out. Tell them he might be blind, but not deaf. Blind, but sober. Blind, but he was going to learn to type and use a computer. Blind, but he was going to get a job again. He wanted to tell them all that, but he didn't. He was just filled with sadness. When Kevin arrived at the Guild, his day turned around. Angel's patience and kindness helped lessen Kevin's anxiety about his dismal computer skills and gave him the encouragement to forge ahead.

Over the next five months, Kevin mastered Microsoft Word and Windows, and he also became proficient in JAWS, a software program that reads text out loud in a monotone, computer-generated voice. JAWS was not an easy skill to master. He'd already spent three hours a day for four months learning to type. As if that was not difficult and time-consuming enough, his JAWS training lasted seven hours a day, Monday through Friday.

JAWS, true to its name, was a treacherous program. Although the user had the ability to regulate the speed, one wrong command, one sloppy keyboard stroke, and what emerged was Latin at best and gibberish at worst. It tolerated zero errors. More difficult yet, the text was read back by a complicated combination of keyboard commands, which changed depending on the computer program being accessed.

With Angel's guidance, however, Kevin became so proficient in his computer skills that he was soon ready for vocational training. Enter Arnie—vocational rehab expert and job placement magician.

Arnie was determined to find Kevin a job, even though he was Arnie's only blind client among the twenty visually impaired people in the group. Arnie had connections with many human resource departments in the city, and the group visited them all. Even though these meetings were pre-arranged, and the organization's company representative understood that Arnie would be bringing a group of disabled prospective employees, finding placements for any of them proved to be a difficult task.

At the end of each meeting, Kevin and the others were invited to ask questions. One exchange at a New York City-based corporation exemplified the extent of the uphill battle they faced.

"Do you remember ever hiring anyone with a disability?" Kevin asked the corporate representative. The woman hosting the meeting pondered Kevin's question for a full minute.

"No, actually," she replied in full candor. "I cannot think of a single one." Kevin feared that he would be among the last in the group to find a job.

The task before Arnie was a difficult one. Yet in the face of these challenges, Arnie was a fierce advocate for all disabled people and determined to succeed. His fellow crusader was Corinne, an anthropologist and sociologist whose professional focus was on improving the quality of life for blind and visually impaired persons.

Arnie and Corinne arranged an interview for Kevin at her agency. A bit of organizational maneuvering on her part produced a position as an intern in her own department. He was employed!

Kevin's first assignment was to assist Corrinne on a project called the "Livable Community Survey" to determine the ten most livable communities for the visually impaired in the U.S. Every day for several months Kevin spoke to numerous visually impaired people around the country asking questions regarding issues such as accessibility at commercial establishments, transportation services, and the existence of sidewalks and their condition. At the conclusion of the survey, Charlotte, North Carolina and Berkeley, California topped the list.

Corinne proved to an advocate for the blind, and a wonderful boss who saw potential in Kevin. She told him that she had set her sights on a professional job for him and began circulating his resume among her many contacts. A combination of her networking and advocacy skills produced Kevin's first professional job since the onset of his blindness. Kevin was grateful for the internship as a transition back into the work force, but this new job felt like hitting the jackpot!

Kevin was hired as a grant writer and researcher. He fully expected to be successful and work for the agency until his retirement. His confidence in his job security was further bolstered when he procured a $2.5-million-dollar grant, one of the largest the agency had ever received.

Sober, gainfully employed, and physically secure once again, Kevin began to relax. His confidence slowly returned. For the first time since the onset of his blindness, he let his guard down, and a crack in his carefully constructed veneer formed.

Light flooded in.

And with it, hope.

SELECTED JOURNAL ENTRY:

July 11, 2015—I'm seeing flashes of brilliant blue light. When it occurs, it is random, yet arresting, and is clearly unrelated to blue-colored objects being present.

CHAPTER 20

Blind Injustice

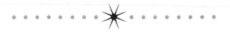

Summer 2002

The beauty of the summer day belied the events that would transpire before sunset.

Kevin was out and about with Ruger and two pals, Sean and Frank. They'd been strolling through Greenwich Village when they decided to stop for a cup of coffee. They walked into a place in the West Village—nothing fancy, just a coffee shop—and waited at the counter to be served.

The young barista noticed Ruger and hurried over.

"No dogs allowed! You're going to have to leave, sir." Kevin was used to this type of encounter, and he was ready with his standard reply.

"He's a guide dog. I'm blind." The young woman either didn't hear him, didn't care, or both.

"No dogs allowed!" Her voice went up an octave. "No dogs allowed!" A restaurant employee who was ignorant of access laws was nothing new to Kevin. He had his follow-up response ready.

"Can I speak to the manager, please?" As Kevin waited patiently for the manager to arrive, another customer approached him at the counter. She stood directly in front of him, but then addressed Frank.

"Does he know what kind of dog this is?"

"It's his dog, why don't you ask him," said Frank with an edge in his voice. The woman repeated her question to Kevin.

"What kind of dog is that?"

"He's a yellow Lab," Kevin replied calmly, despite his increasing irritation.

"Are you sure? He looks more white than yellow to me!"

Kevin was irritated by the stranger inserting herself into the situation. He wanted to say something snarky like, "I'm blind, but maybe you're color-blind!" Just then, the manager appeared.

"How can I help you?"

Kevin took out his wallet and held up the bi-fold card that listed the long-standing legislation that ensured access for guide dogs in public places. The manager took a cursory look and wasted no time in backing up his server.

"That's all very well, but I'm sorry, sir, dogs are not allowed in our restaurant." Kevin proffered the card again.

"Look at it. It lists the access laws that apply to all restaurants," he emphasized. The manager refused to take it from his outstretched hand. He became agitated and abruptly changed tactics.

"You're not blind anyway. You're looking right at me." Frank and Sean couldn't quite believe what they were hearing and tugged on Kevin's sleeve to let him know they wanted to leave. It was clear to Kevin that they had had enough even before they issued their not-so-subtle threat.

"Come on, Kevin. Let's just leave," said Frank. "There's another way to deal with this." Outside, Frank, an attorney, put his hand on Kevin's shoulder.

"No one! Not you, nor anyone else for that matter, should be treated that way! If it's okay with you, I'm going to file a complaint with the New York City Human Rights Commission."

"Fine with me," snorted Kevin.

* * *

Three months later, they were given an appointment at the Commission. The day before, Kevin's friend Adam, a public relations professional, sent out a press release, to Kevin's surprise: "Blind man and his guide dog refused service." The piece was quickly picked up by the Associated Press. In turn, it was distributed throughout the New York metropolitan area to television, radio, and print media outlets.

When Kevin arrived at the Commission's office on Rector Street in lower Manhattan he was accosted by both television and radio reporters shoving microphones in his face. He felt both exhilarated and terrified simultaneously. His first interview was with Magee Hickey of WNBC TV. Next up was Al Jones from 1010 WINS Radio. Over the next several days, the "Ruger Coffee Bar" story was covered on four New York City news programs, two radio stations, and in two newspapers.

Following this barrage of local media coverage, a producer from the *CBS Evening News* contacted Kevin. Equipped with a hidden camera, he recorded Kevin's comings and goings as he and Ruger were ejected from various business establishments throughout the city. The story ran on the *CBS Evening News*; Dan Rather even promoted it during *60 Minutes*.

"Coming up this week," intoned Rather. "Blind injustice, and how many blind Americans are denied service because of their seeing-eye dogs."

Soon after the CBS report aired, a producer at CNN, Vivian Foley, contacted Kevin. Ms. Foley had a different angle for her potential story. Her interest was in how Kevin had learned to live as a blind man in a sighted world. Kevin was happy to be interviewed because he felt that his story might shed a light on the difficulties faced by other blind people living in the city. Ultimately, fourteen hours of videotape were edited down to a four-minute piece.

It opened with Sean verbally describing the Metropolitan Museum of Art's Richard Avedon photography exhibit to Kevin. It then cut to Kevin's other friend, Bill, describing to him Barney's legendary holiday windows.

After footage of Kevin working out and navigating the streets of New York City, the profile concluded with one final dramatic question from the reporter, Michael Oku.

"Is it better to have been born blind, or is it preferable to have had your sight and then lost it?"

Kevin didn't have to think for long about his answer. "I'm very grateful that I was able to see for thirty-six years, and as a result, I have many stored visual memories. It would be very challenging to describe certain concepts to someone who had been born blind, and as a result, had no visual frame of reference." Oku paused at Kevin's response, and then Kevin continued with a question of his own.

"How would you describe the ocean to someone who had never had sight?"

The media coverage was a watershed event in Kevin's ongoing life with blindness. He was gratified that his activism was helping to educate the public about access for guide dogs, as well as, the difficulties for blind people in general. On a personal level, Kevin was pleased to finally feel visible again.

SELECTED JOURNAL ENTRY:

August 22, 2015—my brain is struggling to interpret color once again. I'm wearing a deeply saturated fuchsia shirt, and I can only see the blue pigment that went into creating the color.

CHAPTER 21

Random Acts of Kindness

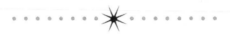

Summer 2003

Kevin was grateful to be employed again, even if the adjustment to being back at work was difficult at first. Soon, however, the benefits began to show. The extra money coming in was welcome, of course, however, having a place to go during the day, and becoming a useful member of society once again were rewards that far exceeded the monetary gain.

Like all of us, Kevin had good days and bad—days when people were kind and days when nothing seemed to go his way. One morning, he set off to work wearing his favorite pair of black suede Ferragamo loafers. As he approached the corner, a kind voice called out to him.

"Hey, careful there! You're about to step into a huge puddle!" Kevin appreciated the stranger's warning. He loved his Ferragamo shoes.

"Thank you!" Kevin exclaimed. The stranger then gently took his elbow and guided him around the puddle to the safety of the dry sidewalk on the other side. The man continued to walk in his direction.

"Do you mind if I walk with you a bit? I'm going this way, too." Kevin was hesitant to say yes. He was not used to strangers speaking to him, nor to random acts of kindness, for that matter. However, he sensed that the man was no threat.

"Sure, but I'm just going to work around the corner, and we're almost there," Kevin replied, to let the stranger know that their encounter would be brief.

"Great," said the man. "Just a little ways then." There were a few moments of awkward silence. Then Kevin's new acquaintance spoke again.

"You weren't always blind, were you?" Kevin wondered how he could possibly know that.

"No. I lost my vision five years ago due to a rare genetic disorder," Kevin explained.

"Oh, wow," replied the man. "I'm so sorry to hear that." While Kevin appreciated his concern, he was far more intrigued by the stranger's apparent knowledge of the timing of his blindness.

"By the way, how did you know I wasn't always blind?"

"I can tell by the way you carry yourself." Kevin had no idea what the man meant by his explanation, but time ran out for a follow-up question. The two approached Kevin's office.

"Well, I'm going in here," Kevin said, motioning with his thumb to the lobby of his building. "Thanks again for saving my favorite pair of shoes!"

"Oh, you're welcome. Have a good day!" Just as Kevin and Ruger were about to enter the revolving doors, he felt the man touch his shoulder.

"I just want you to know that you're a strong man. A really strong man." And as suddenly as he had appeared in Kevin's life, the nameless stranger was gone.

Kevin found his way to the elevator bank and waited for the next car to open. As he entered it, he felt his eyes sting. Without further warning, tears were streaming down his face.

"I am a strong man!" he said to himself, a lump forming in his throat as the truth of the stranger's statement sunk in. "Especially considering what I've been through in these last few years."

After work that evening, Kevin took Ruger out for his final walk of the day. As he bent down on Lexington Avenue to scoop up Ruger's little gift to the sidewalk, he felt a gentle hand on his shoulder—the second that day. This time a woman's voice spoke to him.

"You don't know me; I live in the neighborhood. I see you around all the time." Although Kevin was a bit perplexed as to where this particular conversation was headed, he was polite.

"Yes, I live right here in this building," Kevin replied motioning to his apartment building behind him.

"I know," replied the woman. "I've seen you coming in and out of your lobby for years. I just want to tell you that you are an impressive young man, and that whenever I see you, I have a good day." Kevin felt tears come to his eyes again.

"Thank you very much."

As Kevin walked into his apartment building he realized for the first time that his experience, his daily struggles, had the power to inspire others. On some deep level, Kevin's blindness had a purpose. He sensed that his suffering, and his triumph over it, could help free others from their pain, losses and daily struggles.

As Kevin climbed the three flights of stairs to his apartment, his brain formulated a vague plan of action. He could not have explained it to anyone, or even to himself in coherent sentences. But the outline was there in Kevin's subconscious. It would not only change his life, but many other lives, as well.

A Call to Action had been born.

September 17, 2015—the colors that I can now detect appear as more saturated and less muted.

CHAPTER 22

Words

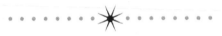

Fall 2004

Kevin knew the power of words.

After the stranger in the street told him he was a strong man, Kevin began to think differently about himself and his life.

As a child, he'd been cut to shreds by the mere utterance of the single word, "fat." Now all it took was to overhear someone say "handicapped."

Although Kevin's self-esteem had been in good shape prior to his blindness, his confidence had taken a serious hit when he lost his sight. Without the bolstering influence of booze, Kevin needed something different to fortify him. The turning point in his search for it came after a party one night.

He shared a cab home with another guest, Juan, who was also returning to the East Side. As they crawled up Sixth Avenue, the street clogged with traffic, Juan told Kevin one "fabulous" story after another about his life. Kevin heard about a holiday spent at a villa in Tuscany, followed by a Robin Leach-like report detailing an extravagant Paris shopping spree. Kevin wondered where all the drivel was leading.

After what seemed like an eternity, Juan informed him that they were nearing Kevin's corner. Not a moment too soon, Kevin thought. Then all at once, Juan grabbed hold of Kevin's hands, placed them in his lap and covered them with his own. Juan then put his face in front of Kevin's and spoke in a hushed tone.

"I need to explain to you why I felt comfortable sharing a cab with you. Back home in Chile, I come from the ruling class, and we were always encouraged by our father to speak to the downtrodden."

Juan's words stunned Kevin into silence. He left the cab shaking his head without saying goodnight. Back in his apartment, Kevin thought about the powerful affect Juan's words had had on him, and he realized that positive words might possibly have the opposite effect. Wayne Dyer's motivational messages and Maya Angelou's persuasive poems had already influenced him. As he took his first baby steps in his transformative journey from anger to gratitude, he had a brainstorm and decided to create his own positive affirmations.

Recently, several friends had mentioned to Kevin that his countenance was serious and stoic, and as a result, he appeared unwelcoming. Inspired by these comments, Kevin decided that his first mantra would be, "I am open and approachable." The results were immediate and noticeable. People began to come up to him on the street routinely, offering help, a warning of impending danger, or simply words of greeting.

Several weeks later, cognizant of the burgeoning success of his mantra, Kevin decided to add several others to his repertoire.

"I am strong, kind, and loving! I am not my blindness."

Again, the effects were startling. After days and weeks of repetition, Kevin felt an inner transformation. A heavy veil of anger was replaced with lightness and warmth. He vowed that he would smile more.

Kevin had begun meditating several years before. He now found himself silently reciting his new affirmations during his meditations. At first, he chastised himself for repeating his mantras rather than focusing on his breathing. He began to feel so much better about himself, and life in general, that he decided not to argue with progress.

In the span of a week, Kevin heard two random people declare that Jack Kornfield had been their conduit into the realm of stillness. Kevin listened to hours of his lectures on Buddhist practice and the transformative nature of meditation. The key to meditation, Kornfield emphasized, was being kind to oneself and free of personal judgment.

His favorite Kornfield message was, "We need to accept that the mind has a mind of its own." This single sentence allowed Kevin to overcome his self-judgment when his mind wandered, and instead to observe the random thoughts and then to return his focus to his breathing.

Within a few weeks, Kornfield's gentle words also taught Kevin that he had the power to acknowledge thoughts about his blindness, and then let them go, as well. The power of words became a crucial new tool in Kevin's efforts to heal his soul. Sober, employed, and happy again, he began the next chapter of his life. What he didn't know, what he could not have believed possible in his most secret dreams, was that the next decade would bring another transformation in his life that neither his doctor nor plain old good luck could fully explain.

SELECTED JOURNAL ENTRY:

October 10, 2015—blisters are appearing all over my forehead, as well as below my right eye. They itch, and as I pop and pick at them, a gritty powder is released. The surrounding area now feels less tight and more alive.

CHAPTER 23

Bumper Cars

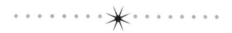

Summer 2005

Summer arrived. The longer daylight hours made little difference in Kevin's muted world. However, he enjoyed shedding winter coats and appreciated the warmth of summer evenings as much as any other New Yorker as he strolled around the city with Ruger. Summer also meant his work organization's annual outing. It was held somewhere different each year, and Kevin always looked forward to it. This would be his fourth one since he began working in the fall of 2001.

This year, the entire staff descended on the amusement park known as Astroland, in Coney Island, Brooklyn. When it opened in 1962, it had a space-age theme. Over the years it had expanded to include rides of every type, speed, and size.

Kevin loved amusement parks, even though he had not visited one since his teenage years. He was excited and determined to go on every single ride at least once, including the Cyclone, a ride he had always feared down to his toes.

The Coney Island Cyclone was one of the few roller coasters in the U.S. made entirely of wood. Its first riders were treated to its historic opening in June 1927. It operated until 1975 when its owners, Dewey and Jerome Albert, entered into an agreement with New York City to take over and operate the ride. It had been refurbished in the winter of 1974 and reopened with appropriate pomp and circumstance the following July. Not much had changed in the ensuing thirty years.

Kevin had the sights and sounds of Coney Island stored away in his memory bank from his last visit. Initially, he was aware only of the sounds: the high-pitched screeching of the sea gulls overhead, as if warning the crowds below, the music of the merry-go-rounds, the laughter, and the excited chatter of children.

Kevin went from ride to ride with a group of colleagues. They began on some of the baby rides and worked their way up. After their fill of the merry-go-round and the Ferris wheel, they headed off to the Cyclone. As Kevin got closer to the front of the line, one of his co-workers, Teresa, noticed he didn't look well. Kevin experienced a vague sense of impending danger and was sweating profusely.

"Hey, are you okay, Kevin?" Teresa asked.

"Yeah, I'm fine," Kevin assured her. "I've been afraid of the Cyclone ever since I was a kid, but I made a promise to myself that I was going on it today."

"Well, it's not written in stone that you have to keep every promise you ever made," Teresa said, with concern in her voice. They inched closer to the point where everyone would be boarding the ride.

"There's still time to get out of line, Kevin. There are four people in front of us. We can come back later if you change your mind." Kevin clenched his fists. He could feel the sweat in his palms.

"Nope, I'm doing this. It's now or never." Kevin had decided that if he could overcome his fear maneuvering the city sidewalks as a blind man, he could overcome his fear of the Cyclone.

The Cyclone stopped and the riders disembarked. The attendant opened the gate to allow the next group in line to enter. Teresa took Kevin's elbow and guided him to their seat, buckled his seat belt, and asked once more if he was going to be all right.

Kevin wasn't at all sure that he was. For a brief moment, he thought he might pass out. The ride took off, and Kevin gripped the safety bar. As the ride mounted its first incline, Kevin's heart pounded in his chest. The ride seem to pause for a moment at the top and then it began its rapid descent. Kevin thought he would be sick. To his amazement, not only was he not afraid, he was enjoying every up and down, every twist and turn.

Unable to see the passing landscape, Kevin was intrepid. He was flying. He was free. His blindness gave him a weird sense of detachment. He could have been in freefall. A man without a parachute. With no visual sense inhibiting his emotions, he enjoyed the speed, the stomach churns, the wind through his hair, and his cheeks billowing in and out, as if made of rubber.

Kevin was alive!

At the end of the ride, he could have gone around again! Buoyed by his newfound confidence, and his determination to go on every single ride at least once, he announced his next destination—the bumper cars. Unable to drive a real car for almost a decade, Kevin decided today was as good a day as any to try out his rusty driving skills.

Seated, buckled in and ready to go, Kevin inched his car forward and gathered speed. Within seconds, his car was smashed into from behind, sending his head whipping backwards and jarring his neck. Before he could regain his composure, another car smashed into him from the side, and Kevin's head was whipped from left to right.

His inability to see was now having the opposite effect. On the Cyclone he had felt free. Here the total lack of control, coupled with not knowing which direction the next blow would come from, was terrifying.

He grabbed his neck and his stomach at the same time. He wasn't at all sure that he could keep from throwing up. As Kevin had no safe way of getting out the car, he had no choice but to endure it. The three-minute ride felt like an eternity. When it was over, Kevin was absolutely done for the day. Nevertheless, he was happy with his achievement. The sudden free falls of the Cyclone were a metaphor for the ups and downs of his life over the last decade. He'd mastered them all, as he had now conquered his childhood nemesis.

SELECTED JOURNAL ENTRY:

November 5, 2015—as I lie in bed, I feel a churning sensation in my upper neck and throat. Strictly on the left side of my face, I feel like blood is flowing, first in the area behind my ear, then in my forehead, and finally, around my nose and below my left eye.

CHAPTER 24

The Christmas Present

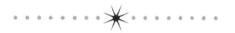

Winter 2008

The next few years passed quietly. Kevin continued to excel at this job, gaining additional grants for his organization. He'd recently landed the biggest multi-year grant his foundation had ever received—a whopping $2.5 million. After many productive years, Kevin assumed that his job was secure. He was, after all, one of the most successful grant writers at the organization.

Kevin enjoyed some discretionary income and was able to afford to treat himself to some new clothes and the occasional meal at a nearby restaurant. Christmas was less than a week away, and Kevin would be spending the vacation with his family at his sister's home in Pennsylvania. He looked forward to giving the presents he had specially purchased for each one of them. As he walked to work that morning with Ruger, Kevin felt an unfamiliar emotion—gratitude.

Something was amiss the moment he walked into the office that cold December day. He felt it on a cellular level, without being able to define exactly what was wrong. He experienced it as a vague, yet certain, feeling that something bad was about to happen.

The morning hours passed quietly. Kevin was distracted by his upcoming Christmas holiday plans. His entire family—all fifteen members—would be there. He was looking forward to spending time with his parents, as well as his sister's two daughters and their families.

After lunch, a colleague knocked on his office door.

"Kevin, there's a mandatory group meeting at three this afternoon in the conference room."

Kevin's vague feeling of unease morphed into a more defined bad feeling. His antennae went up. There was something threatening about the word *mandatory*. Would the group be told that they would not be receiving their year-end Christmas bonuses? Or perhaps next year's merit increases would be delayed? As three o'clock approached, Kevin grew increasingly restless and unsettled.

One by one, the members of Kevin's group assembled in the designated conference room. Sensing apprehension, he imagined the worried expressions and half-frozen smiles in the room. His own anxiety increased with each new person who entered.

His supervisor, the senior VP of development, entered exactly at three o'clock and didn't waste any time announcing her unwelcome Christmas message.

"I'm very sorry to have to deliver this news, especially right before the holidays, but we're experiencing severe financial pressure. Management has enacted some significant cost-savings measures." Stunned silence. The room began to feel close and uncomfortable.

"Among the cost-saving measures is a drastic headcount reduction. I'm sorry but your entire group is being let go, effective immediately," she announced matter-of-factly. Bewildered voices began to ask questions all at once, ranging from issues surrounding severance packages to the possibility of employment in other parts of the organization. The manager did her best to answer them, but the result was the same at the end of the hour-long meeting. All had lost their jobs.

The VP delivered the final blow with the same detachment that she'd delivered the initial news.

"You have until Friday at noon to clear out all your personal belongings from your offices."

Two days!

She left and the group sat speechless. No one moved for ten minutes. Kevin was the first to get up. He returned to his office and started to pack up his personal belongings. A short while later, his immediate supervisor knocked on his door.

"Kevin, we would like you to stay until February to tie up all the loose ends on the upcoming funding reports. Can you do this?"

Kevin was dumbfounded. He'd just been let go without cause, and now he was being asked to work an additional two months. He wanted to say, "No way!" but he nodded his head in agreement and began unpacking again.

Kevin didn't return to his apartment directly from work that evening. He knew that Ruger would be anxious to go home for his dinner, however, he needed to find a support meeting to attend first. His usual one was at seven in the morning before work. Kevin didn't trust himself to wait until the next morning. He was far too upset.

With over four hundred meetings a day in New York City, Kevin knew he would be able to find an evening one. He called a friend who told him of a five o'clock group, just around the corner from his office. Perfect.

Kevin had just finished returning his things to his desk drawers and was getting ready to go when one of his colleagues, Jack, knocked on his door.

"Can you believe this?" he asked.

"Not really," Kevin replied.

"You know, we have until noon on Friday," Jack said. "I'm all packed up. And when I leave tonight I'm not coming back."

Kevin wasn't sure whether he should tell Jack that he'd been asked to stay two extra months. He was still trying to figure out whether this was good news or bad. True, he'd have an extra two months of pay while he was looking for another job. On the other hand, he was pretty sure he'd be miserable working those two months. He also felt guilty having been asked to stay. It would be bad enough knowing that he was on borrowed time; in addition, none of his co-workers would be there to commiserate with over lunch. He considered the possible responses to Jack's statement; then, he decided to tell him the truth.

"They asked me to stay until February to clean up the loose ends on the funding reports."

"Well, of all the nerve," Jack replied. "I hope you told them 'no way'."

Kevin was unable to respond. He settled instead for a simple shake of his head.

"You're a better man than I am, then," Jack grunted. "I would have told the jerks to shove it." With that, Jack left. Kevin could hear him muttering under his breath all the way down the hall. Kevin's blindness was a blessing that day. He was unable to see his friend's faces as he left the building. Still, he could feel their pervasive sadness and worry.

As he walked toward the exit, Kevin imagined cardboard box after cardboard box sitting on dismantled desks, packed to overflowing with the personal items that his friends would be taking home that night. Framed family photos that had adorned their office walls only hours before would be wrapped and placed into flimsy cardboard boxes. He wondered how long it would take his co-workers to find new jobs. He knew that most of them were the primary bread winners for their families. He imagined the gifts and laughter that would be missing this holiday season. Kevin felt sick to his stomach. He also wondered how long it would take a blind man to find another job.

Kevin made the five o'clock meeting with a minute to spare. Although he knew everyone in his morning group, he didn't know anyone that night. Nevertheless, the same warmth permeated the room. So, when it was Kevin's turn to share his story, he poured his heart out.

He told them his sad news of employment, then unemployment, temporary employment, and the prospect of no future employment, all of it happening in just one afternoon. He had a lump in his throat, and the tears came again to his unseeing eyes. He heard a sniffle or two from people seated around him.

Kevin was asked to close the meeting. The compassion in the room as they stood holding hands temporarily lifted him up. In any event, it was time to press on. Ruger was starving and letting Kevin know it.

SELECTED JOURNAL ENTRY:

December 4, 2015—my increasing vision is having a profound effect on how I present myself to the world. The change, although unconscious, is nonetheless striking! My self-conscious, tentative gait has been replaced by a joyous, expansive swagger.

CHAPTER 25

Au Revoir, Ruger

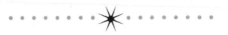

Spring 2008

After Kevin's two-month extension ended, he struggled to find another job. The economy had gone from bad to worse, and even highly-qualified people were unemployed for long periods. Kevin reapplied for his meager disability benefits. Even with the help of his parents, he barely had enough to pay rent. He was also grateful for the generosity of his landlord, who had raised his rent only once in the ten years he'd been living in his apartment.

But Kevin was about to lose something much nearer and more dear to his heart than his job. In some ways, Kevin dreaded this day even more than the one when Dr. Myles had confirmed that his sight was not coming back.

For nine years, Ruger had been Kevin's loyal companion—his lifeline and his best friend in a sometimes brutal world. Whether we like it or not, whether we are ready or not, and whether we can accept it or not, there is indeed a season for all things. And this was the season of Ruger's "retirement." Kevin had put it off as long as possible, but Ruger was having trouble walking and climbing stairs. He knew he had to find Ruger a new home for his final few years. For all his loyal service, Kevin owed him this.

Ruger had received a significant amount of media coverage over the years as a result of Kevin's advocacy efforts. So when it was time for Ruger's retirement, the media was interested in the event. Kevin agreed to record an interview with Trace Gallagher from *Fox News*. The reporter closed with the subject of Ruger's imminent retirement—how he had been Kevin's eyes for the last decade.

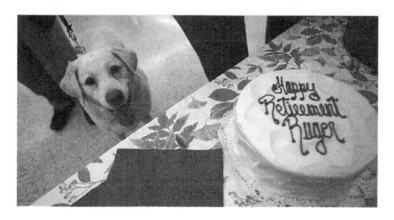

"Kevin, when you lose your sight for the second time in eleven years, how do you say goodbye?" Kevin broke down on camera.

"There aren't going to be any words, just a big hug."

Kevin had been preparing himself for the inevitable day for the last two years. The average working life of a guide dog is seven to eight years. Guide dogs are two years old at the time of their placement. Ruger was now eleven. Kevin heard himself repeating his well-rehearsed mantra on a daily basis. "This is best for him. He needs time to just relax and be a dog. He has arthritis, and he really has trouble with the stairs now." But all the mantras and rational discussions in the world couldn't prepare Kevin for the impending loss.

First, however, there would be one more day for Kevin to spend with Ruger. Friday night, Kevin hosted a party in Ruger's honor in the meeting hall located in the basement of St. Agnes Church. Fifty of Ruger's admirers enjoyed chocolate and carrot cakes adorned with gold icing and blue lettering emblazoned with the sentiment, "Happy Retirement, Ruger."

Ruger, meanwhile, snacked on slices of grilled chicken tossed to him with love by Kevin's friends. This time it was the *New York Times* that covered the event. The party affected everyone present—no one more than Kevin.

Friday night parties always end and Saturday mornings arrive. Kevin and his friend Bob took Ruger to his new home—a thirty-acre farm in Orange County, New York. The owners, Karen and Kurt, were longtime friends of Bob, and he assured Kevin they would provide a loving and comfortable retirement for Ruger. Kevin could not have asked for more.

Karen and Kurt were waiting for their arrival. After lunch, they all took Ruger on a tour of his new, expansive back yard—acres of wooded trails set in a picturesque valley. Kevin reassured himself that Ruger's new home was far superior to the concrete sidewalks that had been his environment for the last decade.

Kevin had designed a careful exit strategy to soften the blow for both Ruger and himself. He bent down and hugged Ruger one last time. He did his best to keep his tears in check because he knew that Ruger would sense them and become agitated. Karen then got Ruger's attention with his dinner bowl and led him into the kitchen for his first meal in his new home.

As Ruger ate his food, Bob and Kevin snuck out the front door. Kevin felt guilty. Like a thief in the night. Even so, he knew he was making the right decision for Ruger. Kevin headed to Bob's car as fast as he could manage without tripping. Once inside, he buckled his seatbelt and collapsed into a torrent of tears.

"I'm sorry," he muttered in between sobs.

"No worries," replied Bob. "I'm having a good cry, too."

For the first time in his life, Kevin felt a crushing loss without the protective buffer of alcohol. Kevin had never before felt such a profound and physically painful emptiness. He had never shed so many tears—not at the break-up of a relationship, not at the death of his grandparents, not at the loss of his job, not even over losing his sight.

Bob started the car and drove away quickly. Kevin had no intention of changing his mind, nevertheless, he was grateful for their quick exit. After an hour of tears, Kevin felt a profound shift, and he unconsciously began to smile. This dramatic change in expression came over him just as suddenly as the crying had. The difference was that now rather than feeling loss, Kevin felt immense gratitude.

Following his blindness, Kevin had feared that he would never experience joy again. Ruger had changed that. He exuded a boundless joy. His lust for life and his in-the-moment exuberance were infectious.

Kevin had felt Ruger's joy. And in the process, he learned to feel his own.

When Kevin returned home, he felt alone. Without Ruger's presence, the apartment seemed empty. Kevin was flooded with memories. First, he remembered Ruger's support when he had stopped drinking—his first recovery meeting with Ruger by his side. He also recalled Ruger's steadfast determination to get him home during the chaos of 9/11—Ruger had been a sea of calm in a city of fear, dust, debris, and chaos. Kevin had been in his computer class on the Upper West Side, and Ruger maneuvered him home through block after block of frightened pedestrians.

Kevin laughed out loud when he remembered the day he had accepted that his initial problems with navigating the city streets and avoiding the omnipresent scaffolding lay with himself, not Ruger. He recalled when his trainer had not spared the full blunt of his observation.

"You're making that dog work for free," he shouted to Kevin. "Praise is his pay check, and he's getting zero from you. Start talking to him right now!"

Kevin recalled one phenomenon, however, that had the power to disrupt Ruger's eternal calm—thunder. During the entire duration of a storm, Ruger was inconsolable. He would sit shaking in the entrance foyer until the storm passed. Nothing Kevin did or said would calm him.

Labradors are known to be water dogs—not Mr. Ruger. Not only did he hate storms, he wasn't that fond of rain either. He would work in the rain, but begrudgingly. In bad weather, Kevin's friends would report that Ruger's characteristically happy face would be overtaken by a frown.

Kevin wondered how he would ever love his next guide dog as much as he loved Ruger. He wondered if Ruger was scared and lonely, too. He'd never met his new people or his new home until that morning. Kevin had not been able to explain to Ruger what was happening, or why. Kevin wondered whether the pain would ever heal.

He thought about his mother's blind friends, Dorothy and Jim, who had recently lost their only son, Michael—an early casualty in the soon-to-be heroin and opioid epidemic that would ravage thousands of promising lives. He was ashamed that he felt sorry for his own loss. How could losing a guide dog compare to the loss of a child?

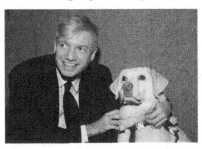

He thought more about Michael's mother who never recovered from his death and would one day return to the solitude of her former calling as a nun, Sister Delores, cloistered in a convent in Pennsylvania.

Because of their early start for the farm, Kevin had missed his prayer and meditation session that morning. He decided to do them that night. Kevin began his meditation on his knees, hands in the prayer position.

He wasn't at all sure he believed that anyone or anything could hear those prayers. Yet he also knew, with absolute certainty, that it was the best, if not only, option he had that night.

Kevin knew he would never see Ruger again. He'd made the painful decision not to visit him because he believed this would be best for Ruger.

"Au revoir, Ruger. You will always be in my heart."

SELECTED JOURNAL ENTRY:

January 25, 2016—throughout my life, I have always seen snow as a nuisance—a hindrance to my mobility. But this morning, as I stroll west on 36th Street, I have an entirely different opinion of it. The snow is the most beautiful I have ever witnessed. It has a striking glow and pearl-essence, as though it is lit from within.

CHAPTER 26

Soufflé and Elias

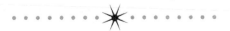

Fall 2008

Kevin was now without a guide dog. Quite apart from the emotional pain he'd felt at having to say goodbye to Ruger, he now had to navigate the streets of New York City with nothing more than his cane. And he still hated it. Reluctant as he was to replace Ruger, it was time to go back to The Seeing Eye.

Because the school named the guide dogs, Kevin was concerned he would get one with a silly name—which even he acknowledged was kind of silly in itself. He'd just heard of two dogs named Browser and Electra.

After a refresher course, Kevin found himself sitting in the Dorothy Eustis lounge once again waiting to meet his new friend. A few moments later, his trainer, Peggy, appeared with a happy-go-lucky Lab who immediately jumped into Kevin's lap.

"Say bonjour to Soufflé!" said Peggy with a laugh.

"Soufflé—really?" Kevin thought, as he shifted in his seat a bit so that Soufflé would get off his lap. Even though she was a mere fifty pounds, that was still a bit too much weight for Kevin to have squirming on his lap. While he welcomed her friendly nature, and did his best to ignore her silly name, Kevin thought that she felt too puppy-like to be a serious guide dog.

Soufflé was a twenty-month-old yellow Lab but much lighter than Ruger who was a sold eighty pounds. Despite her friendly demeanor, as well as her better size for Kevin's New York City apartment, he felt that something wasn't quite right from the moment he met her. Instead of trusting his own intuition and speaking up, he remained silent.

Several weeks later, his training complete, Kevin left with Soufflé determined to make the relationship work. However, right from the start, things did not go well. Soufflé was very needy and wanted to be talked to and petted constantly. She was easily excited and transformed into a gymnast at night, catapulting herself up on to Kevin's bed in an attempt to sleep with him. Old rugged Ruger had been self-sufficient, and Kevin was not accustomed to the extra demands on his time and attention that Soufflé required. Like Ruger, she had a fast pace, and for the most part, was an exceptional guide dog. She managed the stressful city sidewalks like a pro, and for nine months, she performed very well.

The following June, just as Kevin and Soufflé were finishing up their morning two-mile trek, she began to pant rapidly. Kevin assumed she had developed a breathing problem and took her right to the vet for a checkup.

After an extensive physical exam, the doctor gave her a clean bill of health; Kevin wasn't convinced. As soon as he returned to his apartment, he called The Seeing Eye and asked that she be evaluated. Early the next morning, a trainer named Jim came to Kevin's apartment. He examined Soufflé for a few minutes, and then suddenly stopped.

"Is it all right if I take her out for a walk without you?" Jim asked.

"Sure," Kevin replied, although he was a bit surprised by Jim's request. Less than fifteen minutes later, they returned.

"Kevin, I'm sorry, but Soufflé is experiencing an extreme level of anxiety-related panting, and I need to take her out of this environment immediately." Kevin was too dumbstruck and too overcome by emotion to respond. He assumed that Jim would take Soufflé to Morristown for further training and return her within the week.

A special instructor attempted to retrain Soufflé over the next several weeks. She theorized that Soufflé had received an electrical shock from a metal object in the city. Whenever she encountered anything metal, including doors and grates, she would have a panic attack. Jim called Kevin with the bad news.

"I'm very sorry, Kevin, but Soufflé can't work in an urban environment any longer."

Jim explained the special trainer's diagnosis in further detail. That didn't change the facts or make Kevin's loss any easier to accept. Despite their initial challenges, Kevin and Soufflé had become a proficient team. A new void opened in Kevin's life. Once again he was without a guide dog.

The next four months were difficult. After being used to having the benefit of a guide dog, being without one for so long proved challenging. Kevin was grateful that he was proficient with his cane. But a white stick was no match for the expertise, or companionship, of a specially trained guide dog.

Kevin's morning prayers started with a request for another dog that could handle the stress of an urban environment. His specific affirmation was for a strong, steady, and serene companion.

Although he was given priority for a new match, Kevin knew that the pool of guide dogs deemed suitable to work in big cities was limited. Less than fifteen percent of all guide dogs are certified for the demands of a large urban environment. And as was the case with Soufflé, even those who are certified sometimes don't work out.

The call that Kevin had been waiting for finally came in October. He was delighted to learn that a second-generation guide dog instructor, Chris, had been working with the potential candidates himself in New York City for several months, making sure they could handle the extra demands of a big, busy, urban environment.

When Kevin submitted his application for a new guide dog, he'd asked for a male Lab who was strong, steady, and serene. Chris already knew from looking at Kevin's records that Kevin preferred a fast-paced dog, so he'd added that requirement to the list as well.

On Kevin's second day of training, Chris had narrowed his choice down to two dogs. He was having a difficult time selecting between them, and he asked Kevin to prioritize his requirements.

"Kevin, is speed still a critical factor here, or is it more important that the dog is calm?" Kevin didn't have to think long for the answer.

"At this point, speed isn't as important to me as serenity," he answered without hesitation. He then joked, "I'm not such a maniac New Yorker myself these days."

"I think I know what you mean by serenity. We refer to that as soundness."

"Yes, exactly."

"Great!" Then I have the perfect dog for you. His name is Elias, and I've been training him for several months in New York City. The only issue is that his pace is *much* slower than what you're used to."

"Well, that's not a problem then," said Kevin. "We'll go slowly. One step at a time."

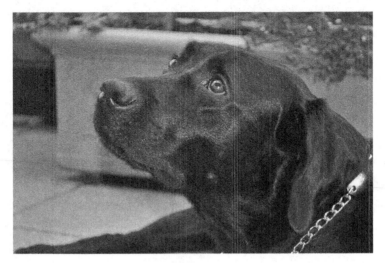

Elias

"Great! He's one of the most beautiful black Labs that I've ever worked with, and I've been training dogs for more than fifteen years. His coat shimmers and his eyes are a deep brown. In fact, I think he really is the most handsome black Lab I've ever seen!"

It was clear that Chris had a big soft spot for Elias. And this was not without good reason. As soon as Kevin met Elias the following day, Kevin knew that Elias was the perfect match.

After two weeks of training in Morristown, Kevin returned to his apartment with Elias. They enjoyed an immediate and strong bond, even though it was an adjustment for Kevin to get used to walking slowly.

Within a few weeks, Kevin realized that Elias was an asset in a way he had not foreseen. Kevin himself was much calmer, kinder, and more serene. Perhaps Elias had his own set of unspoken positive affirmations!

The more time Kevin spent with Elias, the more the serenity that pervaded his nature started to seep into Kevin. It wasn't long before his deep ache for Ruger began to subside. While Ruger would always hold a special place in Kevin's heart, he soon knew that not only was Ruger better off, he was too.

There was one striking similarity that Elias and Ruger shared which helped to keep the memory of Ruger alive in Kevin's heart—nothing could rattle Elias except a good thunderstorm. Unlike Ruger, however, Elias welcomed Kevin's efforts to comfort and calm him until the storm passed. Elias and Kevin settled into an easy routine.

* * *

The next two years passed without further guide dog incidents. However, Kevin remained unemployed. Despite looking every day, he could not find a new job. The market was tighter than ever, and many of Kevin's sighted friends also found themselves unemployed during this time period. Stock and home prices plummeted. The economy went from bad to worse overnight.

Kevin's meager savings were soon exhausted. His social security disability check barely covered his rent. Both he and Elias ate on food stamps. Kevin's protective shield went back up, and he began to pull into himself once again. However, this time Kevin focused on his blessings rather than his losses. He had the sense that Elias was instrumental in his fledgling transformation.

However, what Kevin didn't know was that it would be Elias who would comfort him during the next set of storms that were rapidly approaching.

SELECTED JOURNAL ENTRY:

February 9, 2016—as I lay in bed, I feel a release of pressure, of tightness in my face. The sensation begins in my nose, then directly below both ears, then underneath both eyes. I have the notion that blood is suddenly flowing to areas that had previously been dormant.

CHAPTER 27

Crossing Bridges

Fall 2011

Kevin's father died at the end of the summer. As hard as it was to lose any parent, there had been a significant measure of bittersweet relief for the entire family when Walter passed away. He had suffered a lot in the last two decades of his life following his stroke, and everyone was relieved to see it end.

Selling the family home the year before had been a more difficult transition. Walter was disabled, and Ruth was no longer able to care for herself, much less for him. Kevin's sister, Kathy, found a nice retirement community just ten minutes from her own house in Pennsylvania. It was as perfect as it could be under the circumstances.

Kevin had become attuned to listening to his inner voice. He knew when it was sending him a message, and he paid attention when it did. In the course of one week, he heard two different people share stories about the importance of pursuing one's passion. The first was a self-help writer on Oprah. She espoused the belief that one passionate thing in a person's life can get him or her through any difficult period. The second was a gerontologist (a specialist in the field of aging) who stated that people who live a long and rewarding life pursue hobbies about which they feel passionate.

After the second time he heard the word "passionate" in the same week, Kevin had one of his "aha" moments. He realized that he still had a lot of creative energy that he wasn't tapping into. Years earlier, he had abandoned his photography because he could no longer see the fruits of his efforts. He vowed to himself to do something about that.

Kevin decided that his first step was to keep his ears open even more than usual. The next day, he was struck by something a man said at his support meeting.

"I really love photographing buildings," Jay volunteered to the group when describing a list of things that relieved his stress. Jay was the only person Kevin had ever encountered who also loved photographing buildings. The wheels started spinning in his head. When the group finished, he made a beeline towards Jay.

"Jay, I have a concept buzzing around in my head that I'd like to share with you."

"What's that?"

"Well, we both love photographing structures, and I can no longer do that myself. So would you consider being my eyes and photographing some buildings from my perspective?"

"Sure, that sounds like fun," he replied, an intrigued upturn to his voice. "How would we go about doing it?" Kevin was delighted by Jay's initial enthusiasm and wasted no time launching into his explanation.

"Basically, it would be the two of us trying to capture some subjects I'd had on my list of things to photograph before I lost my vision. I would function as your art director, explaining the angle, lighting condition, and perspective that I would have been looking for with my own viewfinder if I could still see."

Jay loved the idea. He didn't hesitate.

"Let's do it!" Jay shouted with delight.

Kevin and Jay, two men who had hardly spoken until then, were about to become picture-taking partners.

* * *

Two weeks later, on a frigid morning in early December, Kevin and Jay tackled their first project—The Brooklyn Bridge.

The bridge is a hybrid of cable and suspension construction, one of the oldest of either type in the United States. Work began in 1869 with a design by John Augustus Roeblings. Completed in May 1883, it connects Brooklyn and Manhattan, which until then had been separated by the East River.

The bridge was a labor of love for Roebling and one for which he paid with his life. In a freak accident while working on the towers, a ferry pinned his foot against a stone piling. He endured its amputation, leading to a tetanus infection that killed him shortly thereafter.

Roebling was not the only casualty the bridge claimed. Twenty-seven workers died before the construction was completed. His son, Washington, assumed responsibility for the construction during Roebling's disability and following his death. Even he didn't emerge unharmed. Like several other workers, Washington became sick with the bends after ascending too quickly from one of the two floating caissons—giant upside down boxes.

Kevin was thinking about the bridge's opening day as they headed over to Brooklyn that morning. On that May morning, a hundred and fifty thousand people and many ships were present in the East Bay to witness the historic occasion. Kevin felt a sort of opening ceremony was about to take place between Jay and him, as well. Both men set their minds to the task before them as they walked up the weathered, wooden ramp from the Brooklyn side.

"We've got a beautiful sunrise this morning," Jay told Kevin. Suddenly, Jay stopped short and grabbed Kevin's arm.

"Holy shit! The bridge just went from virtual darkness to brilliant light!" he exclaimed with delight. "You were right to insist that we get our butts out of bed early!"

Jay's description of where they were and the surrounding skyline was so thorough that Kevin felt he could almost see it. His heart started beating faster in expectation. He continued his explanation to Jay of the shots he wanted to capture that morning.

"I'm not looking for the traditional poster view of the bridge span. I want to focus on the enormous gothic stone towers that are anchoring the bridge."

"All right," Jay replied. "Let's get a little closer then." When they arrived at the first tower, Jay tugged at Kevin's sleeve. "We're here."

Kevin paused for a moment and took in the smell and sensation of the morning. He could feel the sun rising over the East River and the odor of smoke from the nearby Brooklyn factories starting up their chimneys, as well as the faint aroma of salt from the brackish waters below.

"I want to capture an angled shot looking upward. See if you can get a parallel perspective of the converging lines in your viewfinder," Kevin explained. Kevin heard Jay adjusting the camera's lens. After a few minutes he shouted out in delight.

"I think I have it!"

"Great. Now look for the perspective where there are shadows. I like that better than complete sunlight," Kevin remarked.

Jay found the shots that he thought Kevin wanted.

"Yes, I think I have want you want!"

"Shoot then."

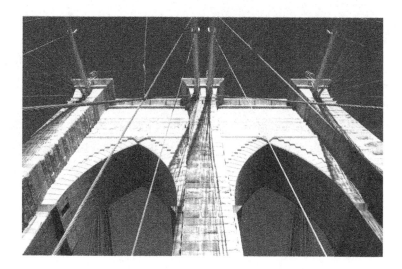

As Jay clicked away, he described each shot that he took. For the first time since he'd become blind, Kevin felt that he was looking through a viewfinder again, composing each photograph, frame-by-frame.

Jay took multiple shots of each tower, as well as the view of the cables—the intricate metal wires that supported the bridge. Each cable was constructed from nineteen separate strands, each of which contained almost three hundred separate wires. In total, there were fourteen thousand miles of wire in the cables.

After several hours, Jay and Kevin decided that they had captured enough shots. They were hungry and getting very cold. As they closed up the equipment, Jay described one last view of the changing light over the Manhattan skyline.

"There's a sort of iridescent, orange glow behind Wall Street now."

"Shoot that too, please," Kevin requested. Then they headed to the nearby subway stop and breakfast.

As Kevin and Jay rode the subway back to Manhattan, they were both physically drained yet exhilarated by their experience: Jay, from Kevin's constant direction and unrelenting questions; Kevin from the sheer delight of finally being able to photograph the bridge from his own perspective.

The following week when Jay described each picture he'd taken, four of the images he had captured were precisely what Kevin had been seeking. However, the most significant bridge Kevin crossed that day was soon to reveal itself, and it would prove to be far more instrumental in his life than even the grandeur of one of the world's most magnificent bridges.

SELECTED JOURNAL ENTRY:

March 3, 2016—I feel a throbbing on the left side of my neck. Thinking it might be critical to increase blood flow throughout my body, I decide to hike the nine flights of stairs in my apartment building two times. The throbbing continues to increase in intensity, as it slowly appears first in the left side of my head, then directly above my right eye. The periodic sensation of first tightness, and then a release, continues for more than two hours.

CHAPTER 28

Itchy Feet

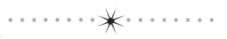

Summer 2013

Kevin got an itch on his left ankle. Then his right. Then both at the same time. A vague discomfort at first, over the next two weeks, the constant itch travelled from his ankles to his toes.

After putting up with it as long as he could stand it, Kevin decided he needed medical help. His dermatologist hadn't heard of anything like this before. A thorough examination revealed nothing on the surface of his skin.

Kevin knew that he was not imagining his discomfort. The questions his doctor asked, in his condescending tone, reminded Kevin of his first inauspicious eye appointment with Dr. Michael sixteen years before.

The doctor did what most doctors would do—he gave Kevin a prescription for antihistamines. After several days of taking them as directed, Kevin was still constantly itchy, even waking up at night.

Then it got worse.

Kevin began to feel a fine powdery substance, a bit like baby powder, being released from his ankles and the soles of his feet. He was befuddled. He decided there was no point in going back to the dermatologist. Instead, he consulted an Ayurveda physician. Under the holistic healing discipline, developed thousands of years ago in India, Kevin's lifestyle, diet, and entire medical history came under scrutiny.

His new doctor explained that when toxins are released from the body, the cleansing process often begins in the feet. This one piece of information was a modest comfort, and he was relieved—if not from the itching, at least from the nagging feeling that he was going nuts.

However, it was Kevin's friend's home remedy, a daily foot bath in dandruff shampoo, which brought him some relief. Then three months after the itching had begun, it just as suddenly stopped.

Then the miracle happened.

* * *

A blanket of humid air covered the streets, avenues, and squares. It was hot. New York City summer hot. Naturally, Kevin's air conditioning chose one of these steamy nights to go on a short vacation.

Kevin slept in fits, tossing and turning until he could no longer stay put. He decided to get up and take a cold shower. He turned the knob and jumped in before he could change his mind. Despite the welcome relief from the heat, the cold water rushing over his head was a shock. Nevertheless, he stayed under the cold stream until he'd cooled down.

He shut off the water and reached for his towel. He stepped out and gave his head and body a good rub down. He decided he might as well brush his teeth since he was wide awake. As he approached the vanity, he stopped short.

A strange light reflected off his bathroom mirror. He thought his mind was playing a trick on him in retaliation for the cold dosing he'd just delivered to his head. He blinked his eyes. He was sure it would no longer be there when he opened them.

But it was. Kevin took his towel and wiped the mirror clean, stood back a few feet, and blinked again.

The light was still there. There was no mistaking it. He wasn't half asleep. He wasn't dreaming. He was seeing a reflection. A few minutes passed. Kevin reached out for the reflection of light; but it had disappeared.

He thought he must have imagined it after all and headed back to bed. He plumped up his pillow and crawled in. He drifted off to sleep, despite the mounting heat and the sounds of the city nightlife outside his open window.

He had a dream. He was a young boy again playing in the open field behind his house. His mother called to him. It was time for dinner. He ran home. He could see.

The next morning Kevin went back to the bathroom and looked toward the vanity mirror. There was only the foggy grayness that had been there for the last sixteen years. There was no sign of what he thought he'd seen the night before.

However, he decided to document it—his first journal entry:

August 14, 2013—entering the bathroom at 1 a.m., I am perplexed and mesmerized by the reflection of light on my medicine cabinet mirror. I think I must be dreaming or imagining it.

Two nights later, he again saw the same light. In the morning, Kevin reached for his journal and made his second entry.

August 16, 2013—entering the bathroom again, I not only can see the light reflecting on the mirror, I can detect a fuzzy outline of a Keith Haring print on the north wall. The image in question is a 12-by-12 graphic depiction of a dancing figure.

Kevin decided to do some more research. Since his blindness had been the result of damage to his optic nerve, he started there. His recent visit to the Ayurveda doctor led him to make a connection between nerve damage and diet.

His initial efforts led him to a study by a British medical group that found a diet rich in antioxidants could promote nerve healing. It wasn't about optic nerves specifically, but *nerves are nerves*, Kevin thought.

Even though he'd begun eating healthier foods a decade earlier, the next day he decided to expand his efforts and added large amounts of foods known to be rich in antioxidant value to his diet—spinach, broccoli, kidney beans, red cabbage, blueberries, cranberries, and walnuts.

While the diet was increasing his daily visits to his bathroom, it wasn't doing much to accelerate the healing of his optic nerve! Still, the antioxidant route seemed to be the only way to go. He thought that maybe he just needed to step it up a couple of notches.

Kevin's further research led him to another website that listed additional foods and spices known to be rich in antioxidants. Cloves, cinnamon and oregano were among the spices noted, but he focused on two others based on gut instinct: turmeric and cayenne.

His research confirmed their potential value. Both turmeric and cayenne have been used for medicinal purposes for thousands of years in India and China. Curcumin is the main active ingredient in turmeric. It is a bioactive substance known for its powerful anti- inflammatory effects, as well as its strong antioxidant value. It neutralizes free radicals and then stimulates the body's own immune system.

Free radicals are molecules that attack cells in the body, causing damage that can lead to diseases. Kevin was drawn to this fact because people affected by LHON are known to have their optic nerves damaged by free radicals.

Curcumin, however, is poorly absorbed into the bloodstream. It helps to consume black pepper with it, which contains piperine, a natural substance that enhances the absorption of curcumin by 2000 percent. Kevin's solution: he began putting a teaspoon of turmeric, along with a few dashes of pepper, into his blueberry yogurt. It was spicy, but Kevin was determined, and a bit of heat at breakfast was a small price to pay.

Cayenne is known to be a circulatory stimulant. It increases the pulse of the lymphatic and digestive systems. In essence, by "heating" the body, the natural process of detoxification is streamlined. Cayenne is what causes people to sweat when they eat spicy food, an important process of detoxification.

While Kevin believed that any healing he might receive would, in large part, be due to grace, there was no doubt in his mind that a significant aspect of it would also rely on his own efforts at detoxification.

Unbroken, undaunted, and now unblinded, Kevin took the next step toward freedom.

SELECTED JOURNAL ENTRY:

April 1, 2016—I'm experiencing pain in my nose, literally between my eyes.

CHAPTER 29

Cheryl's Prayer

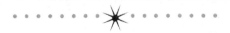

Fall 2013

Kevin's efforts to cleanse his body continued throughout the fall. One day after Thanksgiving, while waiting for the elevator, he was able to see his first written letter in fifteen years.

Kevin recorded the milestone in his journal:

> *November 30, 2013—for several years, I have been able to recognize by touch that there was some kind of sign placed between the pair of elevators on my floor. This morning, as I glance at the sign, I am able to clearly see a bold type black letter A. I can also see that there is smaller type print that I am unable to decipher.*

Kevin had no idea why he was keeping a journal. Nevertheless, he stuck with it, as well as to his diet, meditation and prayers. Despite his Catholic upbringing, Kevin was never a religious person.

That was about to change.

One unusually frigid December morning, the apartment's heating system seemed to be having little effect. Kevin sat on his black leather sofa, shivering. Standing in front of him was a woman he'd just met, Cheryl, who was visiting from California.

She was a friend of Kevin's next-door neighbor, Maria. Several weeks earlier, Kevin had told Maria of the incredible moment when he'd begun to see reflections of light in his bathroom mirror.

Maria was so excited by Kevin's news that she shared it with Cheryl, who was now about to give Kevin his first spiritual healing. Kevin hadn't been too sure of the idea when Maria suggested it, but he figured he had nothing to lose.

Cheryl, like Maria, was a devout Christian and believed in the healing power of prayer. While Kevin continued to shiver, Cheryl began to speak.

"Lord, please heal Kevin's nerves. May they begin to function properly again. In the name of Jesus, surround him with angels. Fill him with your love and grace."

Kevin was uncomfortable at this point, but he stayed put and tried to hide his discomfort. In any event, he was too cold to get up off the couch. Cheryl placed her hands on Kevin's chest, over his heart.

Within seconds, Kevin felt his body flood with an intense warmth. He was shocked, yet he could not deny what he was feeling. The warmth began near Kevin's heart and spread throughout his chest. The lava-like feeling spread up to his neck and down to his waist. Cheryl continued intoning her prayers while the comforting sensation remained in his body for the next fifteen minutes.

From that day forward, Kevin noticed a gradual, but continual, improvement in his vision. While he could not explain what had happened, he believed that either Cheryl's prayers, or her touch, or perhaps both, had stirred up something in his body, as well as in his soul.

* * *

The Christmas holiday officially began the following week. Kevin and his mother went to his sister's house in Pennsylvania. On Christmas morning, Kevin and his mother were in the kitchen alone. The rest of the house was still asleep. Ruth poured herself a cup of black coffee while Kevin sipped on his latest antioxidant concoction—milk and honey. He decided it was the right time to share his miraculous news with his mother. He knew this would be the best Christmas present he could ever give her.

"Mom, I have some really good news to share with you," Kevin began.

"You got another job?" Ruth asked in excitement. It had been five years since Kevin had lost his job, and other than the odd temp job here or there, he'd remained unemployed, subsisting on his meager social security disability check.

"No, Mom, this is even better news." Kevin paused. "Five months ago I started to see a little bit again."

Ruth put her cup down slowly. She tilted her head and glanced sideways at Kevin. Kevin was surprised that he was able to see her do this. Her outline was vague, but Kevin was able to make it out.

"What? What did you say?" Ruth asked in excitement.

"I have started to see again," Kevin answered in a matter-of-fact tone.

With a sweep of her hand, Ruth knocked over her coffee. She ignored it as it dribbled across the table and onto the floor. Kevin explained his story starting at the beginning.

"One night in August when I got up to go to the bathroom, I noticed a reflection of some sort in the mirror. A few days later, the same thing happened again, and that time I was also able to make out the outline of a picture hanging on my wall."

Ruth began to cry. Kevin jumped up from his chair and hugged her. She continued to weep for the next fifteen minutes. Finally, she collected herself and spoke.

"When this happened to you, when you went blind, I thought it was the most tragic thing that could happen to anyone. But it seemed even worse for you, because you were always such a *visual* person." Ruth paused. Kevin waited for his mother to continue.

"You really *saw* everything. You noticed every detail. I'll never forget the time you came to visit when you were living in Washington. You were so upset when you went into the backyard and noticed that our mimosa tree was gone. You were angry with me for letting our next-door neighbor cut it down, even after I explained that the tree's roots were choking off his plumbing. You never believed that, did you?"

Ruth started chuckling. Kevin wasn't sure if it was a result of his news, her memories, or both. He felt the need to temper his mother's joy with a bit of realism.

"Don't get too excited, Mom. I can't see yet. It's just that I am no longer totally blind."

"Ah, never you mind! I know your sight is coming back," Ruth said in delight, and then continued reminiscing. "I also remember how annoyed you were when we got another blue car. You asked me why we couldn't get a silver or white car for a change."

Kevin chuckled, reciting his exact words—blue kitchen, blue house, blue car. His mother seemed so happy that Kevin allowed her to have her moment. He wouldn't rein in her expectations further that morning.

Ruth knew Kevin was not religious in the way she was, nevertheless she interjected some of her traditional beliefs into their conversation.

"I hope you will continue to see more and more, dear. I'm going to pray for a full restoration of your eyesight."

"Thanks, Mom, so will I," Kevin replied surprising himself.

"I know you pray from time to time, and that's good. In addition, it wouldn't hurt you to set a foot or two into church once in a while. You don't even have to attend Mass. You could just light a candle and say a prayer—I know you like Saint Pat's."

While Kevin was anxious to please his mother, and he indeed did like St. Patrick's Cathedral, he was unlikely to ever set a foot in church. Nevertheless, from that Christmas day forward, Kevin wasn't shy to ask his friends, or even strangers, to pray for him. Even the ones he knew might not pray.

"If you don't believe in prayer, no problem," he told them. "Could you just send some positive energy my way, please?"

Kevin could not explain, even to himself, what was happening inside his body. Up until the moment he'd received Cheryl's healing, he'd been somewhat cynical by nature. He'd not been heard to utter the word *gratitude* in public, nor to feel much of it in the privacy of his own heart. However, as the frigid December days ceded their grip to the spring sunshine, despite an upcoming loss that would devastate him, Kevin's attitude toward life shifted from one of detachment and anger to one of acceptance and love.

SELECTED JOURNAL ENTRY:

May 1, 2016—it is so incredible to be able to voluntarily move my eyes once again. However, as I look far left or right, or all the way upward, I feel a strain in my face and neck. The sensation is similar to muscle pain when working out.

CHAPTER 30

One Last Kiss

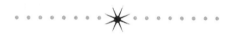

2014

Kevin was relentless in his quest to restore his vision.

It was a cold January morning when he'd first started exercising his eye muscles. They had become weak from nonuse over the last seventeen years. Kevin believed that his eye muscles, while not directly related to his level of sight, were nonetheless still connected to it. He also had a secondary motivation—he knew that his right pupil in particular rested in the outside corner. Kevin was determined to strengthen the muscles so that his pupils would be positioned in the center. While this had the primary benefit of maximizing his sight, it also had a secondary benefit of improving his appearance.

Kevin couldn't help but chuckle when he wondered if he might end up cross-eyed as a result of all the exercises. Even if this were to happen, it was okay with him as long as he could see again!

Kevin's customary time to meditate was four o'clock in the morning. It was the only time the city was quiet, and he relished those first few morning hours before the sun rose. In this relaxed state, he added his eye muscle exercises to his morning routine.

He'd hold the brush in the center of his face. First, he moved it backward and forward directly in front of his nose. Then he repeated the exercise, moving the brush from left to right. Next, at an angle—out to the right, back to center, out to the left, back to center. He forced his eyes to follow the direction of the brush, even though it was only a blurry object in front of his face.

* * *

After nine months of daily exercises, while doing his brush routine one morning, Kevin realized that he could see his fingers. Up until that moment, an object had to be black or very dark for him to recognize it with his central vision—the part that is directly in front of his face.

This new development prompted Kevin to replace his black hairbrush with a flashlight. Kevin started off by repeating the same back and forth, left to right and angled patterns he'd been doing with his brush. Now, he added a new pattern with his LED flashlight pointed at his eyes. He held the flashlight approximately twelve inches in front of his nose. He began by forming a large square in front of his face. He then progressively reduced the size of the square, forcing his eyes to follow the light using his central vision.

After completing a round of progressively smaller squares in a clockwise direction, he would reverse the pattern and do the same set of exercises again in a counter-clockwise motion. To alleviate his boredom, Kevin added new patterns including waves, swirls, hills, valleys and paisleys. Finally, he progressed to the letters u, v, x and z.

Kevin "graduated" to unassisted exercises, rotating his eyes and holding each pose for two minutes. This was not only more difficult but also quite painful, for reasons he was unable to explain. The noon and six o'clock positions came easily. The stubborn three and nine o'clock positions took more effort to master.

Despite the difficulty, Kevin remained positive and committed. His eye muscles had been weakening over two decades, so he knew it would take more than a few exercises to make them strong again.

Kevin was looking forward to Thanksgiving. He was excited to share his additional good news about his eyesight with his family. His sister, Kathy, had arranged to pick him up on the Wednesday before Thanksgiving in the front of his building. As he waited with Elias, he had a strange sense of foreboding that he sought to shake off before she arrived. He decided to take a brisk walk around the block with Elias. Rounding the corner of Lexington Avenue, he heard his sister shout out his name from her car. She had just pulled up in front of his building.

It was perfect timing.

As Kevin and Elias jumped into Kathy's car, he had an inexplicable sense that nothing was perfect after all.

Kevin couldn't wait to be with his mom. He visited her only four times a year, and each visit was precious. For more than forty years, Ruth had been a heavy smoker. The bad habit had finally caught up with her. She was on portable oxygen twenty-four hours a day which made Kevin's conversations with her on the phone difficult.

Ruth had prayed for Kevin every day for the previous sixteen years. In the last year since first learning of Kevin's returning sight, she had prayed even more often with a conviction and vigor that only a mother could have.

Kevin and Kathy drove in silence for the first thirty minutes. At first, Kevin didn't think too much of it since he knew his sister liked to be quiet until she got out of the city. Despite picking Kevin up for his visits for the last seventeen years, she still found the city traffic challenging and needed to concentrate. As soon as they exited the Lincoln Tunnel, she broke the silence.

"Kevin, Mom's doctor called last week to say that she was refusing to take her medications." Kevin felt a slight catch of his breath.

"That doesn't sound good. Mom knows better than that," Kevin said. "I have a feeling that she must know something; she would never refuse her medications without good reason."

Kevin's mother was a retired nurse, and she knew the repercussions of not following the normal dosing regimen of her medications. His sister said nothing and replied with a nod of her head, rather than using words as she had always done since Kevin's blindness.

He saw it. Kevin saw her nod her head!

As soon as they arrived at Kathy's house, Kevin jumped out of the car with an uncustomary lack of caution and went inside to find his mother. She was sitting on the living room couch staring out the window. Kevin went over to her, knelt down at her feet, and gave her a big hug. Ruth smiled. As happy as Kevin was to see his mother, he was also concerned about the news Kathy had shared with him during their ride.

"Mom, Kathy tells me that you are not taking all your medications. Is something wrong?"

"Dear, there is no need to worry. I stopped taking some of them because I don't like the way they make me feel." This seemed like a rational explanation to Kevin. It was late. He decided to let the subject drop for the time being.

The next day was Thanksgiving. The entire family, all fifteen of them except Ruth, had a hand in preparing the meal—Kathy's husband, Tom, made the turkey; Kevin, the stuffing and vegetables; Kathy, the pies. Kathy's grown daughters, Kristin and Kelly, set the table. Ella, one of Kelly's children, had made the place cards.

Kevin heard the Macy's Thanksgiving Day Parade on the TV. He liked this. After the parade, the omnipresent college football games began; Kevin was not interested in any of them, although he never complained.

As usual, Kevin sat at the kitchen island with his mother. Ruth seemed content, though she wasn't behaving like her normal self. She was quiet and restrained. She also didn't make any attempt to interact with Elias—ordinarily, she would have slipped him treats when no one was looking. Even when Kevin could not see her do this, he always heard Elias smacking his lips in appreciation. Of even greater concern was Ruth's lack of interaction with her two great-grandchildren.

Kathy and her girls were busy setting the table. Ruth perked up a bit when dinner was ready.

"It's time to eat!" Kathy announced.

"I'm starving!" Ruth exclaimed. Kevin thought his mother's professed interest in food was a good sign. However, Ruth didn't eat much that night. Kevin was now able to see well enough to notice that while she was busy moving the food around on her plate, very little of it made its way into her mouth. Kevin stayed close to his mother, holding her hand whenever possible.

Everyone finished dessert; it was getting late. The time to take Ruth back to the nursing home arrived too soon for Kevin. He didn't want his mother to go. But Kathy had to make the trip there and back, and Ruth was tired.

Kevin walked out to the garage and helped his mother get situated in the front seat of Kathy's sedan with her seat belt secured around her thin frame. He reached down and gave Ruth a long hug.

"Bye, Mom," Kevin whispered. He then turned around and went back inside the house, wiping away a tear. Just as he heard Kathy's car start up, he felt compelled to go back to the garage and hug and kiss Ruth one more time. He let his gentle grip around his mother's frail body rest just a bit longer than normal.

"I'll call you tomorrow, Mom."

It was to be the last time they spoke in person. Two days later, Kathy called Kevin with the sad news that their mother had died.

SELECTED JOURNAL ENTRY:

June 10, 2016—I'm having a recurrence of something I witnessed before during my healing process. On my forehead, directly to the left of my right eyebrow, I have a feeling of profound tightness. As I touch the surrounding area, I feel blisters that are roughly the size of the head of a pin. If I pick and scratch at them, the tightness is temporarily relieved.

CHAPTER 31

In Focus

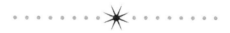

2015

Kevin's mother's death left a void in his life that was impossible to fill. Ruth had been Kevin's staunchest supporter through all his various challenges, from a chubby child to a blind man. However, despite her passing, he still felt his mother's presence as the improvement of his vision accelerated.

Throughout the winter, Kevin had continued his exercises to strengthen his eye muscles. He'd also remained dedicated to his daily prayers and meditation, as well as, to his diet. His positive affirmations were also part of his daily regime.

Kevin was committed to his belief that his eyesight would one day be fully restored. A breakthrough came in May. Kevin walked into his bedroom and found Elias laying on his bed. Nothing unusual about that.

But, Kevin suddenly realized he could see his face! It was the first time he'd ever seen it, and the sight of it brought Kevin to tears. He recorded the unprecedented event in his journal.

May 1, 2015—I glance in the direction of my bed, bathed in afternoon sun and am startled to see for the first time Elias's strikingly handsome face. Tears of joy flow freely. I'm not a crier—but this is a moment that is shaking me to my core.

Kevin's vision continued to improve throughout the summer and fall. He ended the year on a high. Kevin watched his first movie in almost twenty years.

December 27, 2015—I'm watching the Julianne Moore film "Still Alice." It is an intense movie and her performance is phenomenal—but what is important for me is that for the first time in 18 years, I am viewing a movie by myself and am catching virtually every frame. There are a few instances where I am not sure exactly what is happening on the screen, but I am able to deduce that she is looking at a word, either in a book or on her phone. Something as simple as watching a movie is one of those things we all take for granted. Before I lost my vision, I always had. I will never again do that!

However, despite the sight of his beloved dog's face, as well as his first movie, the most important gift Kevin received in 2015 was a complete pivot in his inner focus. He became filled with a joy and a feeling of gratitude that persisted despite his continuing daily struggles.

A few days before New Year's Eve, Kevin fell outside his apartment building on an unexpected pile of trash. Bracing for the fall, Kevin put both hands up in front of him and waited to hit pavement. When he stood up, rather than cursing about the fool that had left piles of discarded moving boxes on the sidewalk, he thought he was lucky that the boxes cushioned his fall such that he didn't break his wrist or rip his new winter jacket!

SELECTED JOURNAL ENTRY:

July 20, 2016—I continue to furiously pace back and forth in the long hallway outside of my apartment. The neighbors may think I'm crazy, but there is a method to my madness. It is clearly helping the nerves to heal. As I walk back and forth, putting pressure on my feet, I feel a sensation in both my neck and spine. Similar to when I got sober, I'm going to any lengths to bring back brilliant clarity and vivid color to my world!

CHAPTER 32

Snowfall

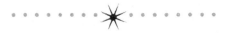

Winter 2016

Kevin had been thinking about this moment for some time. While he had become used to walking without either Elias or a cane, he had never ventured outside without *both* of them. It had been sixteen years since he'd taken a walk by himself. Kevin was always pushing himself to take the next challenge, though, and so he set out one morning in January solo.

He chose a challenging day to do so.

A record-setting blizzard had dumped almost twenty-seven inches of snow on New York City throughout the previous day and night. Kevin knew a cane wouldn't provide the usual tap, tap, tap guide on sidewalks hushed by snow.

His destination—the corner deli—was just two blocks away. He made his way carefully along the first block then stopped short at the crosswalk. An enormous mound of snow lay in his path. It was difficult even for sighted pedestrians to jump over it. Kevin paused. Maybe he should return to his apartment? Suddenly, a man called out.

"Stay put. I'm on my way over. I'll help you cross." A few seconds later, the man was at Kevin's side and took him by the elbow.

"Come this way a few steps. There's a narrow passage through the snow over here." Kevin couldn't believe his luck. His maiden voyage without Elias or his cane, and a Good Samaritan appeared out of nowhere.

"Thanks so much," Kevin said. "I'm just wondering how you knew that I needed help." He didn't think he looked like a blind man these days. The man laughed.

"I'm Hector, the manager of the restaurant across the street from your apartment building. I've been watching you come and go for years, but I've never seen you walking on your own before." Kevin was a customer at the restaurant, and it served one of the most delicious burgers he'd ever eaten.

"What are you doing out here alone, anyway?" Hector asked.

Kevin laughed. "Where should I begin?"

Up until that moment, Kevin had seen snow as a hindrance to his mobility. The snow that day, however, had a far more positive and deeper meaning to him—one that signified his return to independence.

The winter passed slowly. Finally, spring arrived, and when it did, Kevin and Elias returned to the busy New York City sidewalks. Their outings covered several miles each day, without harness or cane. Elias was now simply Kevin's companion.

Kevin woke up on Easter Sunday feeling excited. Despite the morning rain showers, he wanted to go out and shout the news to the world that his sight was improving. He settled instead for his morning meditation and prayers—a routine that he was convinced was instrumental to the miracle he was now experiencing.

After he finished, he tried to interest Elias in a short walk, but he refused. His stubbornness seemed to say, "It's raining. You want to walk? Go for it! I'm staying here!"

Kevin set out alone. At the corner of Lexington and 34th, he ran into a neighbor, Joel, who was taking his two dogs out for their morning constitutional.

"Hey, Kevin, how you doing? It's Joel. Did Elias let you outside by yourself today?" he jested.

Kevin had met Joel a few months earlier, when his dogs had become friends with Elias, as they strolled their Murray Hill neighborhood together. Apart from dog talk, they'd had no real discussion about Kevin's blindness. Still feeling upbeat, Kevin decided this was the day to share his good news with Joel.

"Elias is no longer a guide dog."

"What do you mean?" Kevin replied with a smile.

"I know you've only seen me outside with Elias, but I've been walking by myself since January."

"Wow, that's amazing. Please tell me more!"

"Well, the story actually begins several years ago. I got up in the middle of the night to use the bathroom, and I saw a light. Ever since then, my eyesight has been improving."

"That's awesome!" exclaimed Joel. "I am so happy for you! Are you taking an experimental drug? Did you have an operation?"

"Well, actually, neither."

"So, it just happened? All by itself?" Joel asked, now locked onto what Kevin was saying.

"I started meditating and praying several years ago, and I think that's the primary reason my eyesight started to return. And I also put myself on a strict antioxidant diet," Kevin knew that Joel was an avid meditator and healthy eater himself.

"Oh, I totally believe in the power of meditation and prayer," he said. "In fact, I head up a meditation group at the college where I work as a counselor." Kevin had clearly chosen the right person to share his news with. He continued.

"Even though I was raised Catholic, I never had much of a relationship with God."

"Well, do you believe in a higher power?"

"Yes, I'm convinced there is some form of a higher power, even though I can't describe what that is."

Two weeks later, Kevin ran into Joel again. This time Kevin had some business on his mind.

"Hey, you mentioned that your wife recently published a book. Do you mind asking her if she knows of someone who will write my story for me?"

"That's a great idea," Joel exclaimed. "I'll ask her as soon as I get back to the apartment."

SELECTED JOURNAL ENTRY:

August 1, 2016—my right eye, long behind the progress of the left one, is slowly coming to life. My angle of view continues to increase. Likewise, I feel like it is tracking and following more.

CHAPTER 33

The Yellow Cab

Summer 2016

It was a day for routine matters—the dreaded yearly dentist visit. Not for Kevin, though that would have been bad enough. This was even worse. It was Elias's turn.

Kevin stood on Lexington Avenue in the rain with his hand up. More than one yellow taxi sped by without stopping, even though Kevin had outfitted Elias with his seeing-eye harness that morning. Most drivers didn't want a large black Lab in the back seat of their cabs, guide dog or not.

Especially a large, smelly, wet one!

Kevin was about to give up when a cab finally stopped. He and Elias jumped in the back seat before the driver could change his mind. Within moments, Kevin knew he was in the presence of a positive and powerful energy. It was inexplicable, yet he could feel it emanating toward him from the driver's seat.

After a few moments talking about the crummy weather, the cab driver changed the topic.

"I have a friend back in Russia," he began. "He was nearly blind. He worked with numbers, and he had to hold the ledgers right in front of his eyes to see them. A few years ago, he had a corneal transplant, and now he sees great."

Kevin, for reasons he couldn't quite understand other than the desire to share his joy, decided to tell the driver the abbreviated version of his story.

"Unfortunately, that operation wouldn't help me see better," Kevin replied. "As strange as it sounds, every part of my eye, including the lens, cornea and retina, are all good. It's the optic nerves that are the problem."

"Oh, I'm so sorry," the driver replied. He hesitated as if he was going to say something else, but didn't.

"The good news is," Kevin continued, "three years ago I saw a reflection in my bathroom mirror after seeing nothing at all for sixteen years. Since that day, my vision has slowly become better and better."

Kevin shared more details as the driver continued to listen intently. Before Kevin knew it, the driver pulled up in front of the animal medical center. He jumped out and opened the car door. Kevin paid him, shook his hand and started to walk away. Then he turned back. Something compelled Kevin to make a request.

"Please keep me in your prayers, sir."

Kevin could see the driver's smile. He spoke with an authority Kevin didn't doubt for a second but found almost disconcerting—as if it were coming from another realm.

"That won't be necessary. Your sight is coming back! And trust me, it will be even clearer than before."

As Kevin waited for Elias to be called to the examination room, he replayed his conversation with the taxi driver. Would his sight fully return? Would he indeed be able to see more clearly than before? He spoke out loud, startling the receptionist.

"I will see with crystal clarity!" Now he realized—now he understood—the true and enormous power behind the taxi driver's words.

When Kevin's vision had been 20/20, he'd taken it for granted. But he hadn't seen what was truly important. He'd been an angry man, his attitude toward life making him *blind* to the truth. He drank himself into the haze of blackouts. He saw only a hostile world that wounded him. He saw what was wrong in people, not what was right.

Yes, when his complete vison returned—and it would—it truly would be clearer than ever before. Already, Kevin saw beauty in everything and everyone. He saw the value of the smallest of life's blessings. He had discovered the power of gratitude. He had seen the arrogant and self-absorbed man of his youth fade into obscurity.

With his improving eyesight, Kevin would once again look out at the world, yet his focus would remain steadfastly inward.

To navigate that landscape, Kevin continued to rely on his heart.

SELECTED JOURNAL ENTRY:

September 4, 2016—as I leave my building early this morning, I hesitate as though I can see someone coming in. As I stand still and focus, I realize that I am seeing my own image reflected in the plate glass door as I push it forward.

EPILOGUE

November 9, 2016

Kevin finally agreed to go to the doctor. On the morning of his appointment with a new ophthalmologist on Long Island, he woke up early. His stomach was in knots.

Joel offered to drive him; Kevin was grateful for more than the ride. He was anxious, and he welcomed Joel's company and reassuring words.

The moment they pulled up in front of the office, Kevin began to sweat, despite the crisp fall air. He knew what he could see, but he didn't know what the results of the tests would show. How much of his central vision had returned? He knew that many people affected by LHON learn to function quite well with their peripheral vision. Is that what Kevin was doing? Or did he indeed have some of his central vision restored, as well?

Dr. Richards' assistant was expecting Kevin. The moment he entered the waiting room, she smiled and spoke to him in a cheerful voice.

"Dr. Richards will be with you in just a few moments." Kevin took this as an auspicious sign.

Joel, ever the good Jewish mother, was already thinking about the lunch they would have when they returned to the city. He and Kevin had made plans to meet up with Traci, Joel's wife, later that day.

"Kevin, what do you want for lunch today?" Before Kevin could answer, he was called into the examination room. An hour later, Joel and Kevin were heading back to the city.

They met up with Traci who was waiting for them in front of her apartment. They walked together to a local Italian restaurant. Traci gently took Kevin's arm as they crossed Lexington Avenue.

They entered the restaurant and were shown to a round corner table. The maître d' distributed menus. Kevin didn't pick his up and settled for one of the specials the waiter described. Their salads arrived. As Kevin ate, he noticed that Traci was looking at him.

"What?" he said.

"Well, what did the doctor say?"

Kevin pointed to his mouth full of food, gesturing that he would answer after he swallowed.

When Kevin finished chewing, rather than answer Traci's question, he asked her one instead.

"Are those pearl earrings you're wearing real?"

Traci instinctively reached for her ear lobes.

"Can you see these?" she asked in disbelief.

Kevin's big smile was his answer.

SELECTED JOURNAL ENTRY:

October 4, 2016—I'm walking with a distinct swagger, not one that comes from a place of ego—one that is fueled by immense gratitude and joy.

As he went along, he saw a man blind from birth.
His disciple asked him,
"Rabbi, who sinned, this man or his parents
that he was born blind?"
"Neither this man nor his parents sinned,
but this happened so that the works of God
might be displayed in him."
–JOHN 9

I see God as all love. A spirit that is everything and present in all that is good. From the tiniest life form to the largest scenic landscape and everything in between. I am sure that definition is inadequate, but that is close to what I believe right now.

-KEVIN COUGHLIN

KEVIN TODAY

Kevin remains legally blind. He can't read or drive a car. However, he saw the blue color in the sky in May 2017. The stars in June. And the men's Wimbledon final in July.

However, the main change is the appearance of his face—it appears to radiate or glow. He describes it as a feeling of joy. Some people have referred to it as being connected to their higher selves.

Regardless of the name, the feeling appears to be the same.

Something like grace.

Something like love.

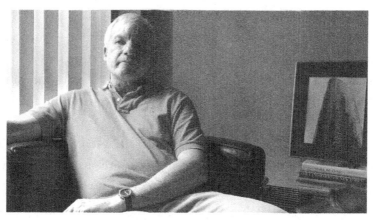

Kevin, May, 2017, NYC.

APPENDIX A

KEVIN'S JOURNAL

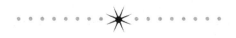

2013

August 14, 2013—entering the bathroom at 1 a.m., I was perplexed and mesmerized by the reflection of light on my medicine cabinet mirror. I thought I must be dreaming or imagining it.

August 16, 2013—in the wee hours of the morning—entering the bathroom again, I not only could see the light reflecting on the mirror, I could detect a fuzzy outline of a Keith Haring print on the north wall. The image in question is a 12-by-12 graphic depiction of a dancing figure.

November 30, 2013—for several years, I had been able to recognize that there was some kind of sign placed between the pair of elevators on my floor. This morning, as I glanced at the sign, I was able to clearly see a bold type black letter A. I could also see that there was smaller type print that I was unable to decipher.

December 23, 2013—having just finished my morning prayer/ meditation, as I reached to turn on Joe and Mika, I could clearly see the contrast of an ivory colored throw on my black leather sofa. It was more than merely the contrast—I could see the waffle-weave pattern of the wool.

December 25, 2013—as I sat having my coffee in the kitchen of my sister's home in Lititz, PA, for the first time I could see a gauzy outline of the granite island where I sat. More striking, I could witness light pouring in from a skylight located in the cathedral ceiling in the great room.

December 31, 2013—pulling a large dinner plate from my pantry—I was struck that for the first time in many, many years, I was able to detect the border of black squares on the crisp white dinner plate. The squares I saw were not saturated black, but a fuzzy gray.

2014

January 2, 2014—as I walked up a snow-covered Lexington Avenue, glancing downward, I could, for the first time, see a fuzzy outline of my beautiful, ebony-colored guide dog, Elias, against a streetscape of stark white snow.

January 6, 2014—on my early morning walk with Elias—I could actually see where his pile of poop was! Oh shucks. I had so loved all these years on my hands and knees, with a plastic bag covering my hand, meticulously feeling around for it.

February 21, 2014—the fog I'm seeing this morning is environmental, rather than the dense, milky fog that had been my ever-present reality. As I was walking with Elias down Lexington on this rainy, London-like, morning, shockingly, I was able to see shapes and figures rushing by. Still no color, but I saw a man walking a large, fluffy haired, black dog. More startling, I felt myself unconsciously ducking to avoid an encounter with an oversized golf umbrella.

February 26, 2014—Rich and I had dinner at Marconi in the neighborhood. The table was lit with a single votive candle. I was not only able to see the white tablecloth and white plates—I was able to easily locate the meatballs on my plate.

March 1, 2014—the entire duration of the blindness, I felt tightness in my neck and upper back. I just accepted it, as I attributed it to the stress of dealing with navigating the world without sight. Over the last few weeks, I had the realization that the long-held stiffness has mysteriously subsided. Not only do I feel a profound lightness throughout my neck and shoulders, I can for the first time in 16 years, freely move my head from side to side, and up and down.

March 10, 2014—each day is like I'm taking baby steps, learning to see again. In the predawn light this morning everything looks brighter and crisper. After pouring my coffee, I caught a glimpse of my Swedish crystal decanters glistening behind me. Holding one of the pieces, as I peered through it, I saw a cloudy image of my fingers. Even without sight, it has continued to be my pattern to face the mirror as I shave. On this day, I could see a milky white reflection of my hand sweeping across my face with the razor.

March 19, 2014—since Saturday evening, my view has been like watching an exceedingly grainy Super 8mm movie. In addition to being grainy, what I see is not completely still, but subtly moving, like the person who took the film was unsteady with the camera.

March 23, 2014—today the flickering home movie perspective has been replaced by steady hues of gray. It is not better or worse, just different. It is, however, immensely disappointing, as I had hoped that the flickering activity was signifying a breakthrough. I've been praying not only for continued patience, but also for the ability to relax in my faith. By that I mean—continuing to strongly believe my vision is being fully restored, while at the same time endeavoring to not scratch and claw until the desired outcome has been achieved.

March 28, 2014—this morning, on a whim, I purchased a single white calla lily. It is hands down my favorite flower, and the subject of many of my photographs. On this day, I was interested to determine if I could see it. After trimming the stem three times, I placed it in a crystal vase which has an organic, undulating rim. And now for the test—as I focused my gaze, in the shadowy light, I first smiled, and then cried softly, as it became apparent that I was (at close range) viewing this strikingly elegant flower with my own eyes.

March 29, 2014—it is a rainy, drizzly day and my vision is the brightest and clearest it has been since this whole process began. At my meeting this morning on 35th Street, to my left, I could see Angela's white shirt and her shoulder length salt and pepper hair. On my right, I could see Rich's dark shirt and his close-cropped grayish hair. Later when I stopped at the Murray Hill Market, for the first time I could see not faces, but figures and body shapes for Diane and Sunny. Diane is thin and petite, Sunny is stockier.

April 8, 2014—once again, I found myself walking in early morning, drizzly fog. What was different today was that walking up 37th Street toward Lexington, I could clearly see gates of brownstones, and stoops bathed in warm light. What I was experiencing, what I was viewing, was remarkably similar to what I recall seeing on this neighborhood route pre-blindness.

April 10, 2014—as I walked up Lexington to my afternoon appointment, I had the realization that in this moment, in bright daylight, for the first time since this whole process began, I was able to see shapes of passersby. Not only could I make out fuzzy shapes of pedestrians, and cars whizzing by, I also had random flashes of clarity. In a momentary flash of light, I glimpsed a shiny belt buckle, a glistening door handle, light bouncing off a screen of a cell phone. Prior to this, in daylight everything was washed out by the sun.

April 14, 2014—today is the first day that my vision appears to be worse. It is gray, blurry, and exceedingly pixilated. However, I feel with every ounce of my being, every cell that something incredible is stirring. My optic nerve is undergoing a gut renovation—a rebirth!

April 15, 2014—my perspective is like a back-lit, overexposed, black and white negative.

April 18, 2014—I feel that I'm on the threshold of a fresh, brilliant new life.

April 20, 2014—for more than three months, I've been religiously viewing the Janet Jackson "Love Will Never Do without You" video on my computer. It is not because I have any affinity for the lyrics; instead, I chose it for my vivid recollection of its circa 1990, striking black and white Herb Ritz photography and art direction. It was my contention that it would be beneficial to exercise my eyes by viewing it, even if I could barely see it. At first, I could just sense subtle movement. With time, the contrast became more pronounced, and I could detect more movement. Today, I could not only follow the choreography, I could clearly see arms, heads, torsos and even fuzzy faces.

April 25, 2014—this morning I awoke to a rerun of the Super-8 movie effect. Today's incarnation is much brighter than previous ones, with more contrast and dimension. That said, it is still disorienting. Images flutter slightly, frame by frame.

April 29, 2014—I'm still experiencing the black and white home-movie effect. Starting this morning, however, there is more pronounced contrast, and I have noticeable depth perception for the first time. Also noteworthy is that I'm seeing stainless steel objects (that had previously manifested as fuzzy white) without the benefit of any overhead light. Standing at my kitchen sink, my eyes unconsciously perused my Dansk tea kettle and Waring blender.

May 1, 2014—the flickering has stopped. It has been replaced by the overexposed black and white negative rerun. Today's incarnation has greater depth and clarity, however. As I was standing in the shower this morning, I was able to view a grid of tiles delineated by white grout.

May 10, 2014—I now consistently have depth of field, and I'm beginning to see weather conditions as they actually are. Yesterday was a cloudy day, and I viewed the day as I recall viewing a cloudy day, pre-blindness. Thursday was a bright sunny day, and even though I was sporting sunglasses, it was still quite bright. This is growth, as I still could see the silhouettes of trees on 36th Street, as well as the cars stuck in traffic.

May 15, 2014—I'm seeing fog for good reason—it is an exceedingly foggy day!

June 2, 2014—last night, at about 5:30, I was walking Elias on Park Avenue. While Elias was busy sniffing a tree, I was standing still facing west. Glancing downward, displayed on the chest of my pink Lacoste shirt, I clearly saw a willowy, shadow of a tree branch shimmering in the late spring sunlight.

June 22, 2014—yesterday morning as I was waiting in front of my building, I saw water flowing from a hose while Omar was watering the plants.

July 11, 2014—since Jimmy Fallon premiered, I've been watching several times a week. Not only is he immensely talented—he repeatedly makes me laugh! I've witnessed incredible progress with my eyesight, as I've watched night after night, kneeling directly in front of my ancient 17-inch Panasonic television. In those early shows, I could merely detect movement of his fuzzy image delivering his monologue. Over time, I could see more detail and greater depth. I could gradually begin to see his hand gestures and hilarious dance moves. As I watched on this night, I could see the outline of his face. Although there was no sharpness to the image I was seeing, I could see the shape and position of his eyes and nose. My perspective at this moment was almost like a charcoal drawing of Fallon's face. Any way you look at it—from nothing to something in three months is extraordinary.

July 21, 2014—patience, prayer and turmeric; the foundation, the corner stones of my journey out of the darkness. Each one of these elements has played a critical role in the process. Since October, in addition to a diet replete in anti-oxidant rich foods, I've been ingesting cayenne pepper and turmeric four times a day. The cayenne I mix in a glass of water; the turmeric is hidden in lemon or blueberry yogurt.

August 1, 2014—as I was deciding which polo shirt to wear, suddenly I was able to see subtle tinges of color. As I held the deep purple one up to my eyes, I saw a whisper of violet. When I examined the vibrant orange one, I saw sand-washed light orange. This is noteworthy, as I've up to this point only seen black, white, shades of gray, and silver.

August 8, 2014—as I was brushing Elias this morning, I saw his eyes for the very first time. They were gleaming ebony, like keys on a Steinway.

August 9, 2014—to measure my progress, I just watched the "Love Will Never Do Without You" video for the umpteenth time. It was strikingly sharper and crisper. For three months, I've been able to see Janet Jackson's dance moves, her arms, head, and back, but was barely able to detect the two featured men. Today, I was able to clearly (in a relative sense) see both Antonio Sabàto, Jr. and Djimon Hounsou.

August 22, 2014—when I woke up last night to go to the bathroom, my vision was like looking directly through the ocean as waves gently roll in. It was not blue like the ocean, but punctuated by various shades of gray. Throughout, there were also random snippets of bright white light.

September 13, 2014—for nearly two weeks, my view of the external environment has changed from one of black, white, and gray to multiple shades of beige. It ranges from a buttery camel to a deep saddle tan.

October 4, 2014—today my view is much brighter. My eyes also seem more open; perhaps more light is getting in.

October 7, 2014—since January, every morning, without fail, I've been exercising my eye muscles by slowly moving a clothes brush in front of my face. The black brush is about five inches long and about three inches wide. First, I slowly move it in the center, lining it up with my nose, back and forth. Then I repeat the practice front left to right, back and forth. Then I proceed, on an angle out to the right; on an angle out to the left; close into my eyes; then further away. Today, as I was putting down the brush, for the first time I could see my finger, about six inches in front of my face. Prior to this, the object had to be black or very dark in color for my eyes to be able to detect it in the center of my visual field.

October 13, 2014—the conventional wisdom is that blind people have a highly developed sense of smell. Well let me dispel that notion once and for all. I never had much of a sense of smell, and it became even worse following an ear infection I suffered at age 20. Nor did it become any more acute following the onset of my blindness. That is, until today—suddenly and dramatically I now have a normal sense of smell. So far today, I've smelt coffee brewing, a bar of soap, onions and a citrus fragrance that I sometimes sport, Lacoste Green.

October 15, 2014—for more than a week, every evening I've been slowly moving a two-inch LED flashlight in front of my eyes. Holding the flashlight in my hand, I pretty much mimic the movements I've been doing with the clothes brush for the last nine months. However, in addition to up and down and side-to-side, I've come up with a new pattern. I begin by forming a large square with the light; then I continue to form smaller squares as my eyes follow closer and closer to the center of my vision. After I've created a series of progressively smaller squares in a clockwise direction, I change direction and form the same light images in a counter-clockwise direction.

October 18, 2014—I caught a whiff of bacon this morning. It smelled glorious!

October 21, 2014—beginning three nights ago, when I've awoken to go to the bathroom, I've felt movement in my neck and spine. The sensation is difficult to describe; it is more than a tingling—but not quite a throbbing.

November 4, 2014—today, I added a new concoction to my recuperative regime; I began drinking honey and milk. Taken together, they form a powerful antioxidant that has been used by many cultures for centuries. As the saying goes—"it couldn't hurt."

November 11, 2014—throughout the duration of my blindness, whenever someone on the street would offer assistance, regardless of whether I was travelling by cane or guide dog, rarely would I ever accept it. Although I would always say thank you, my tone was frequently less than gracious. Either my tone was abrupt—"thanks but I'm fine," or self-righteous—"thank you, but I do this route each and every day." Interestingly enough, now that I'm in less need of help, I'm finally able to accept it. Today, while on a seven-block walk, sporting my long white cane, I accepted help from three separate individuals. First, at 39th and Lexington, a truck was blocking the intersection. As I paused at the curb, the driver got out of the truck, apologized for blocking my way, as he gently took my arm guiding me around his vehicle. On the next block, as I was crossing to the east side of Lexington Avenue, a delivery man, balancing boxes on a rolling cart, yelled out, "Buddy, just take four steps to your right and you'll miss my truck." As I proceeded north on Lexington, fighting back tears of gratitude, a third passerby asked me if I would like to take his arm to cross 41st. As we reached the curb, I thanked him profusely for his kindness. Suddenly flooded with emotion—I had a moment of clarity—I have nothing left to prove.

November 16, 2014—as I've increased the frequency and duration of my flashlight eye-workouts, partly to alleviate the boredom, I've gotten quite creative with the patterns I'm following. No longer content with mundane side-to-side sweeps, ovals and squares, I've branched out into waves, swirls, hills, valleys, and a myriad of both traditional and abstract paisleys. Finally, I form the letters u, v, x, and z.

December 6, 2014—for the last ten days, my vision has been exceedingly bright with very little contrast. It is sometimes punctuated by random flashes of bluish light.

December 14, 2014—I met someone on the street today who had not seen me since May. She told me that my facial expression looked quite different. I asked her to explain. She stated that I looked much lighter and more alive!

December 24, 2014—siting in early morning stillness in my sister's kitchen, I was suddenly flooded with emotion. The tears left me with a profound feeling of both cleansing and clarity. It had taken me more than ten years to make peace with the darkness, to become its friend. Now, I must learn to embrace the light again, and find comfort in it.

2015

January 4, 2015—each evening, as I'm lying in bed, I continue to feel a tingling sensation in my neck and upper chest. At times I experience a gentle throbbing, as well as a warm sensation. These occurrences vary both in intensity and duration, but generally are most pronounced between midnight and 4 a.m.

January 29, 2015—presently, my field of vision is much brighter. Additionally, from time to time, I experience flashes of blue and green.

February 7, 2015—I'm feeling a profound physical lightness throughout my body, but also in my soul. I'm consciously smiling more and more. After years and years of anger and resentment about the loss of my sight, I've recently let all of that negative baggage go. This is going to sound very Oprah, but I do not care, because I am actually feeling it, and living it. I'm allowing myself, for the first time, to experience joy for my journey. I believe with every ounce of my being—that every heartache, each trial, all of the loss, has molded me into who I am today. I'm strong, kind, loving and exceedingly resilient!

February 9, 2015—last night while walking on Park Avenue, Elias and I ran into a friend of his (a black Lab mix named Winnie). Winnie's owner (who I've previously shared my vision journey with) told me that today, my eyes looked more wide-open and brighter.

February 12, 2015—with the aid of a tiny flashlight, I continue to exercise my eye muscles, with the rigor and determination of an Olympic athlete, training for the event of a lifetime. My regimen includes forming circles within circles; squares within squares; vertical and horizontal ovals; triangles; parallelograms; paisleys and complex maize-like creations.

February 20, 2015—I can see the space between the keys on my computer keyboard. I can also see the negative space between the buttons on my Verizon remote. It looks like a vertical grid.

February 25, 2015—my world, long shuttered, is creeping into focus. Yesterday, I allowed myself for the first time to visualize myself joyfully photographing all of the skyscrapers that have been built in the last eighteen years.

February 28, 2015—at night while in bed, the sensation of pins and needles and subtle throbbing continues in my neck and face. These sensations are now enhanced by a soft creaking noise that sounds like tip-toeing over old floor boards.

March 10, 2015—I'm seeing tinges of color in the environment. It is muted, but it is nonetheless, color.

March 12, 2015—it is so gratifying to know that so many people, even those that I do not know well, are rooting for me. I was just riding up in the elevator with a neighbor, Elizabeth. She said, more as a statement than a question, "You could see where the button was, couldn't you?" She went on to say that she was so happy for me, and only wished me the best. Earlier in the day, I ran into an acquaintance, Patrick, who I had not seen in nearly three years. As I shared my vision journey with him, it was clear that he was overjoyed for me. He stated, "Congratulations! I'm so happy for you. This isn't just good news—it is incredible news!"

March 13, 2015—I walked home after getting a haircut at Astor Place this morning. I'm still using my cane, but it was so freeing to almost see my way as I briskly walked up Park Avenue and then headed east on 34th Street.

March 17, 2015—I'm wearing a sweater that is a deep eggplant shade, and I can almost see it! I see it as a slightly lighter purple than it actually is.

March 19, 2015—when I'm standing directly in front of someone, I see their eyes outlined like a black and white negative. I see the oval outline of the eyes as well as the whites, highlighted as though the person were wearing a jet black eyeliner.

March 21, 2015—for the first time, I have some clarity in bright sunlight. It is very sunny, yet I can see Elias, as well as the trees and fences on 36th Street.

March 22, 2015—my sense of hope is audacious—and sustaining.

April 1, 2015—about three days ago, my viewpoint changed from one of a stark contrast between black and white to one of multiple shades of gray. Another development is that I'm having progressively more clarity in bright daylight.

April 3, 2015—I could look into Francine's eyes. They were in black and white, but I could follow them nonetheless.

April 5, 2015—I just heard a quote by Barbara Brown Taylor that struck a nerve: "We want life to be a train ride, and it turns out to be a sailboat."

April 12, 2015—it is clear to me that things are starting to regenerate. There is a gentle tingling in my face, centered below the cheekbones that occurs from time to time throughout the day. At night there is a subtle throbbing in my throat that is accompanied by a noise that varies from a churning sound to something akin to slowly letting air out of a balloon. It is fascinating that I'm literally hearing those long dormant cells struggling to come back to life.

April 23, 2015—watching Jimmy Fallon a couple times a week over the last 14 months, I've witnessed extraordinary changes in my eyesight. Last night as I watched on my brand new 32-inch Samsung, I was able to actually see the facial expressions (in black and white) that Jimmy was making in a segment entitled "Obama's Expressions."

April 28, 2015—yesterday was characterized by intense activity in my head and face. First of all, throughout the day, I felt an unrelenting pain on the left side of my forehead. As I lay in bed, I experienced continual, yet gentle, throbbing throughout my face, but most pronounced directly under my eyes. At one point, around 1 a.m., I felt a build-up of pressure in my left eye, then a release. It was followed by quite a bit of crusty discharge. Suddenly, my eyes feel living—rooted.

May 1, 2015—I glanced in the direction of my bed, bathed in afternoon sun, and was startled to see for the first time Elias's strikingly handsome face. Tears of joy flowed freely. I'm not a crier—but this was a moment that shook me to my core.

May 13, 2015—suddenly, I'm seeing sporadic flashes of color in the environment. As I walked, I caught a random glimpse of the green and navy stripe on Elias's collar. I also caught a brief glimpse of my arm sporting a bright pink polo. Later, I caught a momentary view of the orange V on my Virginia Lacrosse shorts.

May 27, 2015—for more than a week, at night, I've experienced intense pain in the left side of my face. It is evident that long dormant nerves are firing up. The sensation is similar to what I remembered feeling many years ago with an abscessed wisdom tooth.

May 28, 2015—I'm seeing visual snippets of my turquoise-colored polo. The only colors I have not yet been able to see are yellow and pink.

June 8, 2015—for the past week, all of the activity in my face has been centered directly under my eyes. Throughout the night there has been a persistent throbbing and tightness. Several times a day, I've been lubricating my eyes by flushing them with cold water. Periodically there is a sandy discharge from the corners of both eyes.

June 20, 2015—the throbbing feeling in my forehead and under my eyes has continued. I have to believe that it is a noteworthy occurrence, even though there has recently only been just a negligible improvement in my eyesight.

July 4, 2015—I'm just keeping the faith. I continue to eat well, take turmeric, cayenne pepper, milk and honey, and exercise my eye muscles frequently.

July 11, 2015—I'm seeing flashes of brilliant blue light. When it occurs, it is random, yet arresting, and clearly is unrelated to blue colored objects being present.

July 22, 2015—for the last couple of weeks, people have been stopping me on the street inquiring about my apparent improved eyesight. They either say, "Haven't seen you with your beautiful guide dog lately; or tell me what happened?" Last night I was walking Elias on 36th street (just on a leash without a cane in hand). A man with a little terrier tapped me on the shoulder and murmured, "What happened? I've lived in Murray Hill for more than fifteen years, and I've always been amazed at how gracefully you travelled around the neighborhood with your guide dog. Now you seem fine!" I told him about my two-year odyssey of improving sight. He was so filled with joy for me—that I could not help feeling joy myself. When acquaintances and virtual strangers are filled with happiness for me, how can I resist feeling joy myself?

August 5, 2015—I'm consistently seeing orange and green.

August 19, 2015—last night as I glanced out my back window, for the first time in nineteen years, I was able to see the spire of the Empire State Building.

August 22, 2015—my brain is struggling to interpret color once again. I'm wearing a deeply saturated fuchsia shirt, and I see merely the blue pigment that went into creating the color.

September 9, 2015—I'm able to see that I'm wearing a mint green polo shirt. This is noteworthy in that for the first time, I'm able to detect a color that is not deep and rich.

September 17, 2015—the colors that I can detect are appearing as more saturated and less muted.

October 8, 2015—as I walked Elias on Park Avenue, I encountered Dr. Alice, a Murray Hill neighbor for more than twenty years. As usual, she eagerly inquired about the latest development with my vision. As I shared the story about seeing more and more color, she said that I looked different. She stated, "Your eyes are more expressive, and your face is full of life."

October 10, 2015—blisters have been appearing all over my forehead, as well as below my right eye. They itch, and as I pop them and pick at them, a gritty powder is released. The surrounding area now feels less tight, and more alive.

October 12, 2015—affirmations have been a component of my spiritual practice for more than ten years. Early on, they might sound like, "I am not my blindness." or "I am strong, kind and loving." My current refrain is, "I will see clearly as I look directly into people's eyes."

October 18, 2015—with conviction, I continue my affirmations. "I will photograph skyscrapers again! I will see clearly again as I look directly into people's eyes!"

November 5, 2015—as I lay in bed, I felt a churning sensation in my upper neck and throat. It continued for more than an hour, until the sensation suddenly moved to my face. Strictly on the left side of my face, I felt like blood was flowing, first in the area behind my ear, then in my forehead, and finally around my nose and below my left eye.

November 30, 2015—I ran into my neighbor Lori on 36th Street. Lori, who has known me with and without sight, said that today, my eyes look like they are both focusing. In the past she had commented that my left eye looked like it was tracking, but the right appeared to be turned outward into space. Additionally, she paid me a compliment that I have not heard in many, many years—she said, "I hadn't noticed before, that you have pretty eyes."

December 4, 2015—my increasing vision has had a profound effect on how I present myself to the world. The change although unconscious, is nonetheless striking! My self-conscious, tentative gait has been replaced by a joyous, expansive swagger.

December 27, 2015—I just watched the Julianne Moore film, "Still Alice." It was an intense movie and her performance was phenomenal—but what was important for me was that for the first time in 18 years, I viewed a movie by myself and caught virtually every frame. There were a few instances where I was not sure exactly what was happening on the screen, but was soon able to deduce that she was looking at a word, either in a book or on her phone. Something as simple as watching a movie, is one of those things we all take for granted. Before I lost my vision, I always had. I will never again do that!

2016

January 25, 2016—I took Elias for a walk, following the 28-inch snowfall. Throughout my life, I have always seen snow as a nuisance—a hindrance to my mobility. On this evening, as I strolled west on 36th Street, I had an entirely different take. The snow was the most beautiful I had ever witnessed. It had a striking glow and pearl-essence as though it was lit from within.

February 1, 2016—the tingling, throbbing feeling that I've been experiencing for many months in my neck and face has traveled to my chest and spine. The sensation in my spine is most often accompanied by a churning sensation in my central chest area.

February 9, 2016—as I lay in bed, I felt a release of pressure, of tightness in my face. The sensation began in my nose, then directly below both ears, then underneath both eyes. Once again, I had the notion that blood was suddenly flowing to areas that had previously been dormant.

February 13, 2016—for the first time since this whole process began, I'm experiencing pain directly behind both of my eyes. I'm seeing this as a positive sign.

February 20, 2016—the tingling and periodic throbbing sensation continues in my upper chest and lower spine. When it occurs during the evening hours, it is accompanied by a whirring wind-like sound.

March 3, 2016—last night at 10 p.m. I began to feel throbbing on the left side of my neck. Thinking it would be critical to increase blood flow throughout my body, I hiked the nine flights of stairs two times. Afterward, the throbbing continued to increase in intensity, as it slowly appeared first in the left side of my head, then directly above my right eye. The periodic sensation of first tightness, and then a release, continued for more than two hours.

March 7, 2016—throughout the day, I kept running into people that I had not had occasion to encounter in quite some time. In late morning, on Lexington and 38th, I felt a tap, tap on my shoulder. Then I heard Lorna's distinctive British enunciation—"Walking without a dog, or cane—this is extraordinary." As I grasped her hand, she murmured, "I've just run into a miracle." Later in the day, I ran into Tim who mentioned that this morning, he glanced out of his office window and was shocked and thrilled to see me confidently strolling up Lexington Avenue, without the aid of a dog or cane. Outside my deli on 34th and Lexington, I heard Calvin cheerfully stating, "He looks pretty good walking right this way—on his own." Giving me a huge bear hug, he said, "I'm still praying for you, and I never stopped!" All three were filled with joy for me. It felt incredible to allow myself to accept and absorb their joy!

March 9, 2016—for the last 48 hours, my mantra has been: "With joy—I will see spring flowers! With joy—I will see smiling faces!"

March 11, 2016—last night there was a throbbing sensation under both of my eyes, as well as in both of my temples. This feeling continued at varying levels of intensity throughout the evening.

March 12, 2016—the ability to see color globally, rather than merely at close range, appears to be creeping closer to fruition. Today's view of the environment is a muted mix of grays, beiges and taupe, peppered by occasional blips of bright blue.

March 31, 2016—my view has been considerably darker, but most images are appearing better defined. Trees and cars are standing out—their borders appearing like they are sharply highlighted.

April 1, 2016—I've been experiencing pain in my nose, literally between my two eyes.

April 8, 2016—it never fails, whenever I'm discouraged about the progress of my sight, I run into someone who has been rooting for me, or praying for me. This morning, as I crossed 34th Street, I heard Calvin's booming voice, "It's so good to see Kevin heading this way, no cane or dog." He shook my hand, saying, "It's coming soon." Later I was stopped by Alan from the neighborhood. "You're looking great, keep doing what you are doing." Knowing how much both of them are pulling for me buoyed my spirits.

April 10, 2016—I just ran into a neighbor walking his dog, Roxy. He stopped, and said that he can tell that I'm seeing better by the way I'm walking.

April 11, 2016—there was an emotional comfort in being blind. There was routine and certainty. In contrast, as my sight has been slowly returning, what I see often varies from day to day. At times it is very bright, other times extremely dark, or lots of contrast, or little if any contrast. Some days, I can see color at close range, or strictly black and white. Still other times, I see hundreds of shades and permutations of grays, beiges, and taupe.

April 13, 2016—last night as I lay in bed, there was intense activity in the area of my face and neck. First there was a tingling sensation just below the surface of the skin, then a feeling of blood flowing throughout my face and neck. This tingle then flow continued periodically keeping me awake for more than two hours.

April 16, 2016—I'm seeing shadows in bright sunlight. As I walked with Elias, I just saw shadows virtually every step I took; shadows of scaffolding; shadows of low fences around trees; shadows cast by parking meters; shadows cast by overhead awnings; shadows created from parked cars. This is striking, previously, as this process has unfolded, the only shadows that I've been able to detect have always been in low light or shaded environments.

April 19, 2016—yesterday, walking on Park Avenue, an Italian tourist attempted to get my attention by saying, "Please sir. Please sir." As I focused my eyes downward, his intention became clear. He was holding a camera, and pointing to his face. Overcome with emotion, I responded, as I pointed to my eyes, telling him, "I'm sorry, but I don't see too well." At that moment, nothing would have given me more pleasure then to be able to photograph that man flanked by Grand Central Terminal.

April 21, 2016—as I continue on this twisting and turning path toward full resumption of my vision, it has become clear to me that seeing is not merely an unconscious act. Instead, it requires an enormous amount of attention and volition. At times I realize that I can actually see something if I just directly focus my gaze on it. Likewise, I've learned that in other situations, if I just look upward, or to my left or right, I can see more and more.

April 22, 2016—once again last night, I experienced a sensation of loosening of tension—of tightness in my neck. What was different this time was that for the first time the feeling was in the front of my neck, rather than the back. On the upper right side of my neck, directly below my chin, repeatedly, I felt the sensation of release, then flow.

April 23, 2016—the daily ritual of doing exercises to strengthen my eye muscles is finally showing some dividends. Until yesterday, if I desired to look up or down, or to the left or right, I had to literally move my head in that direction. Now, I can stand in place, with perfect posture, and with my eye muscles look downward, upward, or focus my gaze to the left or the right.

May 1, 2016—it is so incredible to be able to voluntarily move my eyes once again. However, as I look far left or right, or all the way upward, I feel a strain in my face and neck. The sensation is similar to muscle pain when working out.

May 4, 2016—this morning as I sat in prayer and meditation mode, I began a new eye exercise. I looked to the far left and held that position for about two minutes, then I moved my gaze upward in a clockwise position about 30 degrees and held that position for a couple of minutes. I continued this process in 30-degree intervals until I completed the full circle of my visual field. Picturing the orientation of a clock, I felt the most strain, as well as loudest creaking noise, as I paused my gaze at the 9 and 3 positions.

May 14, 2016—as I walked with Elias on 37th Street, I ran into Joel walking Ellie. He immediately said that my eyes were really moving and following today.

May 16, 2016—as I walked up Lexington Avenue, I just had an experience that I cannot recall ever having before—I saw shadows within shadows, within shadows. In brilliant sunlight, on the sidewalk in front of me, I viewed the shadow of an awning, overlaid with the shadow of a truck, overlaid with a shadow of a tree branch blowing in the wind.

May 17, 2016—periodically throughout my day, I continue to work the nerves in my neck and face by doing the "stare and hold that pose" exercise; proceeding clockwise 30 degrees, focusing and holding that gaze for two minutes.

June 10, 2016—I've had a recurrence of something I've witnessed before during my healing process. On my forehead, directly to the left of my right eyebrow, I've had a feeling of profound tightness. As I touch the surrounding area, I feel blisters that are roughly the size of the head of a pin. As I pick and scratch at them, the tightness is temporarily relieved. Then the blisters reoccur, and I continue the process of popping them.

June 17, 2016—early this morning, 4:45 to be exact, I found myself seated in a wicker rocker facing Lake Mahopac. The delicious stillness was suddenly interrupted by spasms of joy-filled tears. After a momentary lapse, in a split second, my brain caught up with my emotions, as it became evident why I was crying. For the first time in 19 years, I was seeing a star-filled sky.

June 28, 2016—for ten days, tiny blisters have once again been appearing on my skin. This time they have been centered on my right eye. As they appear, I feel an intense tightness. Once I pick at them, the pressure is released. It then feels like blood is flowing in that area.

July 7, 2016—today I began repeatedly cleansing my skin with witch hazel. Initially I was just focusing on the area of my face where the blisters had been forming. Then I realized that I should also apply the witch hazel on my neck, legs and feet, as they are also areas where healing is taking place.

July 10, 2016—for more than a week, I've been clad in my Birkenstock sandals (my most comfortable shoes) as I pace up and down the hallway outside of my apartment. For some reason, putting pressure on my feet and walking appears to be stimulating the nerves in my neck. It actually feels like something in my neck is loosening and breaking up.

July 15, 2016—this morning, I can almost identify items in my refrigerator by sight. For example, the Chock-Full-of-Nuts label on the coffee can.

July 20, 2016—I continue to furiously pace back and forth in the long hallway outside of my apartment. The neighbors may think I'm crazy, but there is a method to my madness. It is clearly helping the nerves to heal. As I walk back and forth, putting pressure on my feet as I do, I feel a sensation in both my neck and spine. Similar to when I got sober, I'm going to any lengths to bring back brilliant clarity and vivid color to my world!

July 28, 2016— this morning as I walked with Elias on 36th Street, a kind voice called out. "You're doing so well! I've seen you on this block for many years. I've wanted to approach you to ask you what has been happening, but I didn't know how to." I introduced myself and asked her name. I briefly told her what has been happening over the preceding three years, and Sondra said that she was so happy for me. As we said goodbye, she said, "My husband has dementia, and your story gives me so much hope."

July 29, 2016—as I continue to walk up and down, putting pressure on my feet as I do, I feel activity in my neck and face. I repeatedly feel a loosening of tightness throughout my neck and face, as well as the sensation of blood flowing to areas that previously had little feeling.

July 31, 2016—I've stepped up the pace of my daily affirmations. My favorite is "With joy, I will look into people's eyes. I will see in vivid color with brilliant clarity." Sometimes, I do the quick version—vivid color; brilliant clarity."

August 1, 2016—my right eye, long behind the progress of the left one, is slowly coming to life. My angle of view continues to increase. Likewise, I feel like it is tracking and following more.

August 8, 2016—I'm able to make out images (in muted shades of beiges and grays) on the television from four feet away. Last week, I had to be directly in front of it, to decipher anything.

August 21, 2016—I feel that blood is flowing above, and around my right eye. Perhaps, this signifies that long dead zone is finally coming to life.

August 25, 2016—in a world hyper-focused on instant gratification, my sustaining affirmation continues to be that old, trite saying—all good things come to those who wait.

August 30, 2016—I feel considerable tingling just below the surface of my face. It is my belief that toxins are also exiting through my skin as well. To help the process along, I'm exfoliating my face daily.

August 31, 2016—as Elias sniffed joyfully on 36th Street, I was suddenly flooded with emotion. After reflecting for a moment, it came to me—the reason why Elias is so special to me can be explained by one word—gratitude. Each of my other dogs were just as important to me, however, back then, I did not appreciate them. I failed to see what was right in front of me.

September 2, 2016—I'm experiencing an intense, recurring pain, deep within the recesses of my nose.

September 4, 2016—as I exited my building early this morning, I hesitated as though I could see someone coming in. As I stood still and focused, I realized that I was seeing my own image reflected in the plate glass door as I pushed it forward.

September 8, 2016—in addition to the pain that is centered deep within my nasal cavity, I periodically have pain throughout my neck.

It is similar to the nose pain in that it emanates from deep within the center of my neck.

September 14, 2016—I ran into Dr. Alice, walking her new puppy, a golden doodle named Gracie. Once again, her kindness and positive energy lifted my lagging spirits. First she said, "Everyone in the neighborhood sees you and comments on how well you're doing." As she hugged me she said, "You're looking wonderful. You are such an inspiration!

September 15, 2016—my reverberating affirmation for more than a week, has been—UNBLINDED will be a # 1 New York Times Best Seller!

September 16, 2016—as I waited on line at my nearest deli, the customer in front of me said, I'm so surprised to see you walking on your own. I asked him if he knew me from the neighborhood. He said that he worked in the building across the street and has seen me around for years. I then introduced myself, shook Tony's hand and shared the brief version of my returning sight. Tony was overwhelmed with joy for me!

September 18, 2016—I continue to feel strongly that the critical connection for my ultimate nerve healing is deep within my neck. At times, it feels like something is breaking up, and other times like something is coming to life.

September 21, 2016—prior to the blindness, and for quite a while afterward, I was self-absorbed, angry and aloof. Today, I am kind, empathetic and serene.

September 26, 2016—last night I felt an itching sensation, and a tingling around both of my eyes. It was different from anything I've previously experienced.

October 1, 2016—I'm experiencing pain in several locations: left side of my head; throughout my face; deep within my neck. I believe that this pain is heralding the renaissance of all of my nerves.

October 4, 2016—I'm walking with a distinct swagger, not one that comes from a place of ego—one that is fueled by immense gratitude and joy.

October 14, 2016—I'm seeing at greater distances. As I walked with Elias this morning, I was struck that as I proceeded eastward on 37th toward Lexington, I could see cars flowing down Lexington Avenue, from nearly 100 feet away.

October 20, 2016—it used to make me livid when I detected that people were talking about me in my presence. No more. As I walked up Park Avenue, I overheard this: "Do you know what's up with that man? Didn't he used to be blind?" Today, I did not engage. I just smiled!

October 27, 2016—for the past week I've had periodic pain throughout my head. The exact location varies, but it's frequently toward the front, directly above my forehead. Today it is very intense.

October 28, 2016—as I sat doing my morning eye exercises, I was startled by quite an unusual noise emanating from deep within my neck. It is my contention that much of the current healing is centered in my neck. The sound was akin to the one heard when hands quickly run over bubble wrap.

November 19, 2016—this afternoon without any precipitating event the left side of my face swelled up. The entire area from just below my left eye to my chin was ballooned out. There was no pain or throbbing—just intense itching.

November 20, 2016—the swelling and intense itching just below the surface of my face lasted for three days.

November 23, 2016—I arrived at my sister's new home in Pennsylvania for Thanksgiving. For the first time in nearly twenty years, I oriented myself to a new space visually, rather than by creating a floor plan in my head.

November 24, 2016—at the dinner table I could clearly see everyone in my immediate sight (up to four feet away)—I could actually see

Elmer to my right, George and Jere to my left. This is striking, noting that last year when Thanksgiving dinner was served at my sister's former home—all I could see then was the contrast of the white electrical outlet cover against the forest green wall.

November 25, 2016—for the last two days I've been experiencing intense throbbing and periodic pain in my spine. When I exert pressure on the area by leaning against the granite kitchen island, the sensation is somewhat relieved.

December 4, 2016—I continue to walk back and forth barefoot in the hall outside of my apartment. As crazy as it might sound, as I put pressure on the soles of my feet as I purposely step—I feel tingling in my neck and spine. This is one of the many seemingly unconventional tools that are collectively bringing all of my nerves to life.

December 10, 2016—often times it feels as though there is some sort of blockage deep within my throat that is trying to unblock. Sometimes I experience extended periods of a yawning sensation—but it is unrelated to being tired. Rather, it is like some function deep within my throat is attempting to fire up. To aid in this process I've been cleansing my throat by gargling with vinegar and baking soda and holding it in that spot for several minutes.

December 17, 2016—watching Elias sniff and romp about in the fresh fallen snow gave me enormous joy! Now hours later, as I reflect on his child-like enthusiasm, I'm smiling broadly.

December 20, 2016—for the last four days I've had itching throughout my head and neck. It is much more severe during the nighttime hours.

December 22, 2016—I've been kept awake the last two nights by intense throbbing in my head and neck.

December 25, 2016—at the Christmas dinner table, I could see on my left as far as Kelly; on my right as far as Tom. My view was considerably clearer and several feet further than it was from the same location on Thanksgiving.

December 27, 2016—the intense itching is continuing in my head and face. It is most pronounced in my face deep under my cheekbones and nose.

Also by Traci Medford-Rosow
Inflection Point—War and Sacrifice in
Corporate America

PROLOGUE
EXCERPT FROM
INFLECTION POINT

New York City, March 13, 2013

It was one of those things you know in your gut long before your brain can register what your eyes are seeing. At first, we both tried to explain it away, but before the day was over, the truth of what had happened to us was unimaginable, yet undeniable.

Peter Richardson, my law partner and long-term colleague and friend, and I were walking back to our office after lunch at one of our favorite little French bistros in midtown Manhattan when he called my attention to a young woman in front of us.

"Look at those pants!"

It was, I think, the first time in the three decades we had been working together that he had called my attention to someone on the street—not that you could miss her. She looked like Lisbeth Salander, the title character in *The Girl with the Dragon Tattoo*, except instead of black leather, nose rings, and tattoos, she was wearing the most outrageous pair of psychedelic pants I'd seen since the hippie '60s. They were neon-bright, a kaleidoscope of colliding colors: swirls of purple, yellow, red, and green striking a bold contrast to the gray overcast of the March sky.

Impossible to miss.

So the very last thing either of us thought at that moment was that she was a spy. Especially since she was in front of us rather than behind.

"Wow, those are bright," I replied. "But sort of a nice throwback."

Thinking nothing further of the woman or her pants, we continued on our way. Two blocks farther south, we stopped at the drug store to pick up a prescription. The normal ten-minute wait at the pharmacy ran a little longer than usual; a quarter hour later, back on Third Avenue, we were heading downtown to our office on East 37th Street.

And there she was again.

She'd evidently stopped to read her BlackBerry. I still didn't think too much of it then—I too have been known to stand on the street reading emails—but it was March, still winter, and still cold, and I remember that it crossed my mind that she must have been into one hell of an email exchange.

Late for an afternoon conference call, Peter and I hurried by the young woman in the psychedelic pants. Four blocks farther south, we turned right, and leaving behind the bustle of Third Avenue we entered the quiet residential side street where our office was located in the commercial space of a Murray Hill townhouse.

We loved our little office and our two-man law firm. It was a totally different world from the one we'd spent in Big Pharma, each occupying those spacious corner offices with dazzling city views. But we were happy in the simplicity of our new world, with our few clients, and even with the extra responsibility that came with not having any assistants to help us with our daily work. Ours had become a small world, unhurried by corporate deadlines and unstressed by corporate bureaucracy.

Once inside our office, we realized that we'd left the case folder on the subject of our afternoon conference call in my apartment, a block away. So, less than a minute after we'd arrived, we were racing out of the office. And there she was, again, standing just a few feet past our door, to all appearances, still texting. My antennae went into full alert.

"Holy shit!" I exclaimed.

We both stopped dead in our tracks.

I looked at Peter; Peter looked at me.

I knew we were both thinking the same thing but were unable to comprehend that we were beholding that same pair of unusual psychedelic pants in the heart of midtown Manhattan for the third time in less than twenty minutes.

"Peter, what are the odds that she just happened to be standing outside the drug store when we left and now just happens to be standing outside our office?"

"Not very high. I think we're being followed," he replied with a sigh. "But, why?"

"I have no idea, but forget that! I'm going to follow her," I said and took off.

Her back was to me, but almost as if she had seen me coming after her, she started to run. She approached the corner where, without breaking stride, she turned her head around and looked at me. Our eyes locked for a split second. I was expecting her to turn left and continue south downtown when she abruptly turned right and headed back uptown in the same direction from which she'd just come, quickening her pace in the process. I followed suit.

At the next corner, she bolted across the street on the diagonal into four lanes of rapidly approaching traffic on Lexington Avenue, all the while looking at me over her shoulder. No sooner had she hit the sidewalk on the other side when she darted back across the street again, accelerating into a full-out sprint. Breathless, and with my mouth open, I stood on the sidewalk and watched her disappear. There was no way my old body could keep pace with a twenty-something year old.

After the shock wore off, I went to my apartment and called Peter.

"I'd like to think we are simply very popular, but there is only one explanation I can think of for us being followed," I said and related the details of my further adventure.

"No doubt about it," he agreed with my unspoken conclusion. "And now we've blown our conference call to boot," Peter added, always the pragmatist between the two of us.

"Someone had to have been behind us feeding her information," I said, returning our conversation to the mysterious woman. "That is the only logical explanation for how she knew I'd taken off after her, and why she had turned her head around to look at me."

"Do you think this is the first time, or have we been followed before?" Peter asked, now clearly upset at what had become undeniable.

"No clue."

Peter and I were now retired from Pfizer. We had both worked over thirty years for the company in the legal division, and we'd been involved in a lot of high-profile litigation over the years, including the Lipitor patent infringement case and its settlement.

"And I'm guessing it's the same outfit that hacked into my computer," I said, remembering the unwelcome visitor I'd found scrolling through my *Inflection Point* files in the middle of the night the month before.

I'd been up late, unable to sleep, and had decided to pick off a few emails. Someone had suddenly taken over my computer, in much the same way a remote tech does when fixing it, and the cursor had started moving on its own. I held my breath as my eyes followed the cursor to the left side of my monitor, to my personal folders, where it scrolled down until it found my book's file. That was about as much intrusion as I was able to manage. I started hitting the keyboard at random to make the intruder aware of my presence. In an instant, the control of the cursor was returned to me, and the mysterious interloper vanished into cyberspace. I wondered whether I had chased off the intruder in time, however—before they'd found my secret folder. Their cursor had been close to it.

I couldn't be sure.

"It must have something to do with that Lipitor case," I repeated to Peter in suspended disbelief.

"I can't think of any other explanation," he agreed.

For the next few weeks we both felt uneasy. Was our office being bugged? Were we being watched and followed on a routine basis? We found ourselves looking under our desks and behind picture frames for the telltale signs of little cameras or microphones. We were unnerved when we noticed parked cars with casually waiting drivers outside our apartments, and for a period of time our otherwise ordinary life took on a cloak-and-dagger feel. We became agitated when we saw a strange, camera-like object hanging in the garden at the rear of the house next door to our office. It appeared to be pointed toward our windows. A few days later, it disappeared. We never learned what it was, who had put it there or why.

Winter was at last giving way to the arrival of spring that end-of-March day when I sat at my desk, lost in thought. With the flowers came the first signs of new life, of hope, of a fresh beginning. I wondered whether I'd ever arrive at my own new beginning, if I'd ever get past the journey that had begun for me over a decade earlier on that cold, snowy January morning. I wondered whether the downward spiral of my life would ever reach the upward curve of the inflection point.

Here we go again...

About The Authors

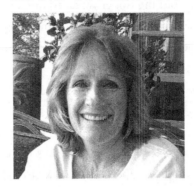

Traci Medford-Rosow

Traci Medford-Rosow is an award-winning author of the Amazon bestseller, *Inflection Point: War and Sacrifice in Corporate America*. She is also the author of *Data Exclusivity* and numerous op-eds published by *Pharmaceutical Executive*.

Traci is a partner in the New York City law firm, Richardson & Rosow. Previously, she worked at Pfizer for thirty years as Senior VP and Chief Intellectual Property Counsel, Global Head of IP Litigation and General Counsel of Europe. She is the founder of The College Education Milestone Foundation, a not-for-profit organization dedicated to helping high-performing students attend college.

Traci lives in New York City and Mahopac, New York with her husband. They have two adult children.

Contact Traci at www.tracimedfordrosow.com

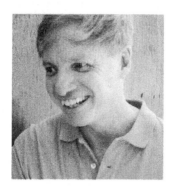

Kevin Coughlin

Kevin Coughlin has appeared on numerous radio and TV shows. He inspired a CNN story chronicling his experience living as a blind person in New York City which was instrumental in establishing its first blind advocacy program. His story, *Blind Injustice*, was featured on the CBS evening news. He lives in New York City with his beloved dog, Elias.

Contact Kevin at www.kevincoughlinunblinded.com

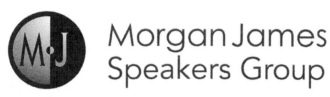

Morgan James
Speakers Group

↗ www.TheMorganJamesSpeakersGroup.com

We connect Morgan James published
authors with live and online events
and audiences who will benefit
from their expertise.

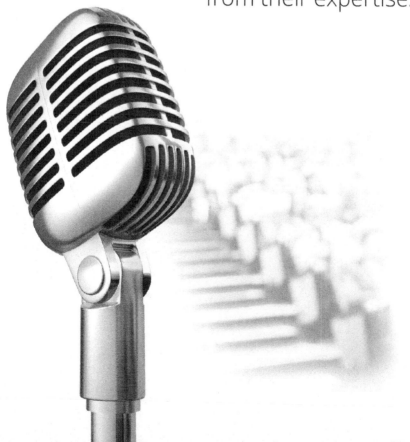

Morgan James makes all of our titles available
through the Library for All Charity Organization.

www.LibraryForAll.org

CPSIA information can be obtained
at www.ICGtesting.com
Printed in the USA
BVOW08s1031140218

508134BV00001B/74/P